Mind-The Basics

By
Kamal Artin, MD

The purpose of "Mind-The Basics" is to inform the public about the basics of psychiatric evaluation and treatment. It is also a simplified source for students who plan to specialize in psychiatry. In other words it suggests minding the basics of the mind to those interested in the field.

Table of content

3

Foreword

I left my homeland where liberty, justice, and equality were not much valued. I left in search of a place, where people's rights and choices were respected and where there was a greater opportunity for progress. I ended up in Switzerland first and in the United States later. After a few years of survival work and learning new languages, I questioned where I fit best in terms of a career. Before beginning my education, I took a questionnaire to see where I best fit in in terms of my career. My answers reflected my interest in the human body and mind as well as the impact of society and culture on ones behavior. This combination of interest convinced me to become a physician in general and a psychiatrist in particular. Thanks to the supportive grant and scholarship by Dr. Brassel, a remarkable humanist at the University of Zurich, I started medical school.

While some subjects were more challenging, my highest grades were often in psychiatry during medical school. I chose the field, did a dissertation in psychiatry in Zurich, and assisted in two research projects on mood disorders in San Diego. Subsequently I was accepted to a few schools such as the University of Zurich as a medical student, the University of California in San Diego as an intern, Johns Hopkins University as a resident, and the University of Southern California as faculty member. I learned a tremendous amount from these great academic institutions and their faculties and am grateful for what I learned from them.

While every one of my mentors deserves much appreciation, my highest regard is for the psychiatry faculty members of Johns Hopkins University especially Dr. Treisman, who immediately welcomed me to the program upon the first interview. I am also grateful to Dr. McHugh and Dr. Slaveny, who with their high expectations and deep understanding about the field became great mentors to me at Hopkins.

I am grateful to Dr. Alan J. Romanoski, for his supervising and editing the case of psychogenic vomiting, to Mrs. Cynthia Rupe for grammatical editing of the book, and to Mrs. Carol Ann Boo for providing the image of the cover.

I am thankful to my friends, and colleagues, and patients who have been a great source of my learning throughout life.

My special thanks goes to my wife and my two sons for their patience with me, without whom I cannot do much let alone write a book.

What I am writing about the mind is based on what I learned from "The Perspective of Psychiatry" by Dr. McHugh and Dr. Slaveny. Of course, one cannot always rely on one's memory and therefore if there are errors in what I state here, only I am to blame. I can claim, "I know no English". I'd rather publish my understanding of the mind simplified for now, while I rely on my memory and opinion, and add some relevant literature review for a few cases. My goal is to share what I believe I know about the mind with the public in general, and with medical students and psychiatry residents in particular.

Psychiatrist, The Physician

Psychiatrists are physicians whose expertise is the assessment and treatment of the mind. Upon completion of medical school, a psychiatrist obtains a specialty degree in mental health from a credible academic institution. Part of this specialty is general training in medicine and focusing on the mind becomes their specialty. Unlike other physicians who might work with tangible, objective and measurable maladies, a psychiatrist's job is working with something that is intangible – the mind, which exists nowhere but in the brain. So one might wonder what differentiates a psychiatrist from other specialists such as neurologists, neurosurgeons, psychologists, and social workers that deal with the brain or one of its products, the mind.

As brain experts, neurosurgeons and neurologists recognize a problem in the brain and its nervous system, such as a tumor, seizures and paralysis. However, these specialists leave the recognition and treatment of the intangible product of the brain - the mind - for psychiatrists, psychologists and social workers. The psychiatrists, who serve as physicians, relate the challenges of the mind to a behavioral, personality, social and/or medical issue, while psychologists and social workers are trained in understanding and treating the first three issues of the mind, but not the medical one. Psychologists focus on and treat various challenges of the mind ranging from personality traits such as impulsivity and shyness, to behavioral actions such as violence and isolation. Social workers focus on challenges of the mind that arise from social, legal and economic issues.

The Mind

In general, the mind is not an easily tangible part of brain function. The brain is responsible for regulating every function of our existence, whether it is breathing, seeing, hearing, sensing, moving, reproducing, eating, drinking, feeling, thinking, etc. Most functions of the body and brain are tangible and measurable with tools available to the medical field. For example neurologists may detect, measure, and treat disorders of strength, sensitivity, movements and memory. Neurosurgeons can do the same for brain mass or bleeding, ophthalmologists for the vision, and cardiologists for the heart. However, if a patient is suffering in terms of feeling, thinking and behavior and there is no obvious medical explanation for the degree of suffering, then it is the job of a psychiatrist to figure out what is happening in the patient's mind via their emotions, cognition, and action.

A simplified analogy of the brain-mind is the hardware-software of a computer. The capacity of the hardware is predetermined in terms of set values such as memory and speed. What software programs add to the hardware is similar to the experiences one gains throughout life. The human brain as the most developed mammalian brain is equipped with the mind, which consists of feeling, thinking and behavior. Lack of basic needs such as food, thirst and sex might make mammals feel afraid, sad, or angry. To meet those needs, mammals think and make a plan. Once they act on the plan they have engaged in a behavior. In contrast to other mammals, the human brain and, therefore, the human mind are more developed. Not only basic needs, but also more advanced needs such as power, wealth and beauty have been added to the humans' list. And with it, a more advanced process has developed in our brain, which has led to a more advanced thinking that includes calculating, planning, convincing, or even lying. The action required to meet these needs has also become more sophisticated, so humans use various tools in their behavior.

Emotion is the way we feel, such as feelings of happiness, sadness, nervousness, and anger. Cognition is how we think and includes the content and the process of our thought. Action is what we do or do not do, as well as intentional or unintentional behaviors. Are changes in feeling, thinking, and behavior normal? Of course, they are as normal as our growth. We do not feel, think, and behave the same in one day, let alone throughout our life. However, a lack or an excessive amount of feeling, thinking and behavior could be a sign of abnormality, in the same way lack of growth or excessive growth is also abnormal.

Feeling

Feeling is the product of a more primitive part of the brain. It can be categorized in four types: happy, sad, angry or anxious. Any other description of our feeling is somehow related to those four types of emotions. For example, if we say we feel mad, irritated, annoyed or frustrated, we mean we are angry. If we feel bad, disappointed, hopeless, helpless or torn, we mean we are sad. Feeling nervous, frightened, scared, worried and concerned are descriptors for being anxious. And when we say we are feeling great, joyful and pleased we are describe a feeling of being happy. An average amount of any of those feelings is necessary for human existence just as an average amount of blood pressure and sugar in the blood is necessary for our survival. It's completely normal to be nervous when facing a new challenge in life. It is normal for a pilot to worry about the passengers; it's normal for a physician to be concerned about patients; it's normal for a mother to be scared about a baby's well being. Furthermore, why shouldn't we be angry if someone takes advantage of us? It is often justified to be frustrated with red tape and bureaucracy. If the frequent nagging of a spouse does not annoy us, then something is wrong with us. And who doesn't get sad with the loss of a loved one? Isn't it normal to be disappointed, if we lose the value of our investments? How about betrayal by a person we trusted? How could we not be happy if we are healthy, receive love, respect or money, or recover from an illness. In short, it is normal to have any of the feelings we experience, as long as it is not excessive and dysfunctional. Persistently feeling sad, down, low, bad, miserable, mad, angry, irritated, confused, lost, on top of the world, anxious, worried, nervous and scared may lead to subsequent negative thinking and actions, and therefore manifest as an emotional disorder.

Thinking

Thinking, if undisturbed, is based on reason. It has a process and content. Its process could be fast, slow, or, in extreme dementia, probably almost gone and, in more extreme forms such as a coma, most likely nonexistent. Its content could be positive and include the greatest ideas about life, philosophy and science. It may also be negative and contain ideas about destruction, violence, pity, suicide and obsession. It is created by the outer and frontal part of the brain and differentiates humans from other mammals, which, proportionally, have a smaller brain size. The frontal lobe regulates decision-making that is triggered by feelings, which arise from a central part of the brain such as the amygdala. Thinking that is disorganized, loose, slow, fast or bizarre, or one that contains hallucinations, delusions, obsessions, suicidal and homicidal ideas, or poor memory or concentration may lead to a disorder of thought and decision making that leads to subsequent actions of significant negative consequences.

Behavior (as a component of the mind)

The behavior is what one does or stops doing. It may be the manifestation of beautiful feelings that leads to a constructive thinking which in turn may be expressed in the form of new discoveries, writing, art, singing and painting. It may also be a manifestation of frustration and hateful feelings that leads to less constructive thinking such as obsession and even destructive thinking and subsequently actions such a violence, suicide or even war. Among the three component of the mind, it's the behavior that is easier to modify. It's for that reason that most mental health centers are called behavioral centers. One might not be able to control how they feel, or stop thinking about certain ideas, and it's absolutely fine to have any feelings and thoughts, even unethical ones. But what is not acceptable is to act out on those feelings and thoughts. It is part of depression to see oneself as worthless and think about suicide, but committing it is not acceptable. Opposing one's foes does not justify homicide. It's fine to feel hopeless and think about getting rich by robbing a bank, but doing it is not acceptable. If behavioral disorders such as impulsivity, compulsivity, violence, avoidance, dramatization and bizarre acting are not changed, they lead to significant negative consequences for the individual actors and people around them.

Normal-Abnormal and Evolutionary Purpose

People who seek psychiatric help usually have difficulty with their mind. Ideally, those who have recognized or been led to recognize that there is something abnormal with the way they feel and think may seek help from psychiatrists before they engage in a behavior. The psychiatrist could lead them to a modified or even positive behavior in such a case. As an example, some may think the best way to overcome a constant anxious feeling is to intoxicate themselves with alcohol or drugs; some may be done with feeling sad and constantly think about suicide; some might have an extreme urge to act out sexually regardless of who they have sex with; some might be angry with the power and wealth of others and think about stealing or destruction of their property. In those cases, a psychiatrist could prevent a negative outcome and encourage such individuals to engage in behaviors that are of benefit to themselves and others. Others will have already acted out with negative behaviors and will come to seek help to prevent further acting out, which is still a positive step. Unfortunately, some never seek help and engage in behaviors that could be harmful to themselves or others. Those who seek help for their feeling, thinking and behavior are evaluated. The psychiatrist determines based on the information provided and obtained that one has an unusual life experience, character, behavior or disease, or a combination of those. Based on the determination or diagnosis, the psychiatrist then recommends a treatment plan.

If a body or mind function is out of order, then it is fair to call it "disordered". It's normal to have blood pressure in the arteries, and sugar and fat in the blood; however, if these are excessive, persistent and recurrent, then the condition is called high blood pressure; diabetes, and hyperlipidemia respectively.

This concept applies to mental conditions too. Everyone has changes in their feeling, thinking and behavior. Those changes are considered a disorder if they are excessive and exaggerated, continuous, create dissatisfaction in life, lead to self-destructive behavior and an inability to function, and disturb social interactions. The disorder doesn't recognize social status, gender, ethnicity or other factors. Abraham Lincoln, who is said to have suffered from a mood disorder, once said: "I am now the most miserable man living. Whether I shall ever be better I cannot tell; I awfully forebode I shall not. To remain as I am is impossible; I must die or be better."

One might argue that there is an evolutionary reason for various human traits and conditions. Mania might be necessary in a primitive society when one has to take care of acres of farmland at a fast pace in a short amount of time. But in a modern society, the consequences of a manic episode could lead to fast and erratic driving, accidents, financial ruin, sexually transmitted diseases (STDs), and even death.

Ironically manic episodes end up with depression. Is it possible that depression and its symptoms such as lethargy and sleepiness after mania are necessary for rest, recovery, and preparation for the next productive manic episode? Depression might lead to loss of appetite, malnutrition, dehydration, and subsequently a seizure. In turn a seizure might lead to recovery from depression. Interestingly we have now learned that a small seizure brought about by ECT is an effective treatment for depression.

It might be necessary for a society to have energetic, aggressive and powerful people to fight as soldiers and defend the community in case of threat. The same applies for other members of the society that are compassionate, caring, selfless and helpful to all, which might be the case in highly spiritual and moralistic people. If everyone is the same in the society, it would be like having a world with only one type of plant or one type of animal, which is impossible for survival.

Reasons behind the Disorders of the Mind

Major psychiatric disorders include: mood disorders, anxiety disorders, sleep disorders, developmental disorders, mental retardation, cognitive disorders, psychotic disorders, adjustment disorders, somatoform disorder, dissociative disorders, factitious disorders, impulse disorders, personality disorders, eating disorders, substance use disorders, disorders during childhood and disorders during late adulthood.

These disorders are mixed in terms of categorization based on DSM (Diagnostic and Statistical Manuel). Based on Dr. McHugh and Dr. Slaveny's perspective at Johns Hopkins University, the factors that make people have difficulty with their feeling, thinking and behavior are diseases, personality, life story and behavior.

Disease

Disease or illness is a condition that a person has or has developed. It is not a choice but an affliction. It means a part of the body from the cellular to the organ level is not functioning the way it's supposed to. When the cells of the pancreas are defective in terms of insulin production, a person has diabetes. There are many clear and objective signs as well as tools that help physicians of various specialties diagnose eczema, hypertension, kidney failure, cirrhosis, muscular dystrophy, arthritis, paralysis, cataracts, endometriosis, prostate enlargement, colitis, cancer and other illnesses. Mind specialists are limited in terms of having tools to diagnose diseases of the mind. They must mostly rely on signs of illness. If a person episodically and recurrently becomes elated, impulsive, loud, promiscuous and/or overly generous, the psychiatrist sees the signs of mania. Persistent sadness along with diminished motivation, energy, concentration, appetite and/or desire leads to a diagnosis of depressions. Frequent and excessive nervousness, restlessness, worry, and avoidance of daily activities (such as grocery shopping) because of fear are signs of anxiety. Being withdrawn, detached from the real world, hearing voices no one else hears, seeing objects no one else sees, and a preoccupation with the belief that one is being followed without any substantive evidence indicates that one has psychosis.

As mentioned earlier, psychiatrists don't have many tools to diagnose an illness of the mind aside from measuring attention, memory, serotonin levels and brain images. However, those measurements are not specific in the same way that blood pressure is measured. There are some reasonable theories about so-called chemical imbalance or imbalance of neurotransmitters in the brain. Imagine for a moment that the brain is a factory with thousands of wheels, each turning another to make a product. For the factory to work smoothly, the wheels need to be oiled properly, otherwise there is potential for squeaking in the wheels and the eventual mechanical breakdown of the entire factory. In the case of too much oil, there might be a mess in the factory that ruins the product.

If the brain cells are the wheels, neurotransmitters are the oil. There is some evidence that with depression there is a lack of serotonin, norepinephrine, or dopamine between the connecting nerve cells, or too much dopamine, in the case of mania or psychosis. Lack of gamma amino butyric acid or increased norepinephrine are the likely causes of anxiety. The factory director's job is to make sure the wheels have sufficient oil to function and prevent breakage and dysfunction so a product is produced. Similarly, the role of the psychiatrist is to make sure the nerve cells have the adequate amount of neurotransmitter in the right balance and place for the brain to function and give a proper product of feeling, thinking and behavior.

If the wheels are organized and turn smoothly, they lead to a purposeful action, the way smooth and properly functioning brain cells communicate with each other. If disorganized, the cells cannot function properly and it may lead to noise, breakage and dysfunction, leading to a mind disorder.

The treatment for any chemical imbalance in the brain is medicine. Antidepressants, anti-manic, anti-psychotic, and anti-anxiety medications were invented based on the theory of chemical or neurotransmitter imbalance. With the discovery of various medications for the mind, millions of people have become able to function as they are supposed to. Of course medications are not risk free, but, overall, their benefit has outweighed their risk (similar to how the benefit of using a car outweighs the risk of a car accident). Some argue that there is a natural way of treating mental illness. However, purely natural treatment could be likened to taking a walk or riding a horse to travel to a foreign country, rather than traveling by car or plane. You may arrive at a similar place, but it may take months or years longer to get there and the risk of suffering and death is higher. It is fine to walk to a nearby grocery store; but it is irrational not take a plane if the distance is too far, despite the minimal risk of a potential crash. The same can be applied to the degree of mental illness. If one has little sadness, it should be fine to use exercise, good diet or some safe natural remedies to feel better. But if one is so severely depressed that life has no meaning, it will be extremely unreasonable, not to mention unethical, to prevent that individual from trying medication. When traveling a short distance, riding a bike or a horse maybe is reasonable. In this same way, one medication to treat mild depression maybe is enough. However, some people need more than one medication for the condition. Most major illnesses are not curable but treatable, whether it is diabetes, cystic fibrosis, or congestive heart failure, symptoms are often managed instead of removed altogether. Similar, there is no cure for major mental illnesses such as depression, mania and psychosis. Fortunately, these major illnesses are treatable and treatment reduces suffering, prevents worsening and makes life better. To maintain a proper level of health and happiness, the treatment of major illnesses should be continued without interruption.

At the same time there are illnesses that are curable, such as various infections, the flu and benign tumors; which once treated, do not need continued treatment. The same argument could be made for some mental disorders. Mild anxiety and panic, a low-grade single-episode of depression, bereavement and adjustment disorder are examples of conditions that with a temporary treatment could be resolved.

In the past, many patients with serious mental illness continued to suffer by receiving only talk therapy. Now many patients receive ongoing medication for less-serious conditions that might not be necessary. This is why evaluation and reevaluation by the doctor and cooperation from the patient is the key. To have such a relationship, the doctor should find a window to the patient's soul. The "window" could be a common interest in activities, a piece of art or a movie they like, a life philosophy, or a place they've visited. Or it could perhaps be a new discovery about life and certain lessons or values the patient shares with the doctor or vice-versa. Once such a window is created, trust is established. However, patient's disappointment, and inflexibility and neglect of the opened window from the doctor, without opening a new one, could lead to interruption of the patient-doctor relationship.

Personality

Personality is what one is. The traits of one's personality or character are usually identifiable and predictable. Most people have a variety of traits that are in balance. Some people may lack certain traits or have too much of others that present as characteristics in need of guidance or treatment. Certain traits we may all have include: shyness, avoidance, worry, withdrawal, impulsivity, gregariousness, recklessness, being too quick to react, slow decision making, being overly-dramatic, being self-centered, clumsiness, honesty, gullibility, determination, flexibility, rigidity, stubbornness, being cooperative, excited, uninterested, suspicious, eccentric, over-dramatic or self-centered, to name a few. No one is perfect and we all have good or bad traits and it does not necessarily matter which ones we have. However, if we have excess or a lack of some critical human traits, we might fall in trouble.

Even certain negative traits may be beneficial for our survival. It is the setting, position or condition we are in that makes our traits helpful or useless, or perhaps even harmful. If five people with a different trait such as being dramatic, impulsive, aggressive, shy, and indecisive are in a jungle and confront a hungry lion suddenly, it will most likely be the impulsive one who makes the decision to attack the lion or run away. If he survives, others will too. However, it is also the impulsive risk-taker who could have been killed first by the lion, which may leave after his hunger, is satisfied without hurting the others. We can't expect an army general not to be suspicious of enemies or not to think aggressively when in war. We cannot expect a priest not to be compassionate and do everything possible to create peace. We cannot expect a shy person to be the master of ceremonies of a party, but he or she can be a remarkable librarian or scientist in a laboratory. We cannot expect a mother not to be full of love and even dramatic and cry when her baby is suffering from an illness. We cannot expect a politician to be dishonest and self-centered while the goal of the person is serving others. It is not unusual for a singer or actor to be self-centered and enjoy the admiration of performing well. A pilot or a physician needs some degree of caution to properly take care of the passengers or patients, respectively. A clumsy person would most likely not make a good surgeon. A person who is gregarious and cunning would do better in sales and marketing than in a scientific laboratory. The same marketer has a better chance of convincing a gullible person than a suspicious one. A gullible person who is selfless and willing to help everyone is a valuable community member when facing a natural or manmade disaster.

However, imagine a person has many traits that are negative such as recklessness, impulsivity, dishonesty, self-centeredness, and compulsive lying. Such a person likely has a disorder that could cause problems for the patient and others, therefore requiring treatment. The same applies to a person who is shy, withdrawn, indecisive, and is overly-dependent would likely miss much in life and deserves to be guided with therapy to overcome their weaknesses. The purpose of treatment of a personality disorder is not to change the person, but to make them aware of their strengths and weaknesses. Treatment is meant to help and guide the individual in finding the setting that is suitable for growth and development, and practice constructive behaviors while avoiding destructive ones. Medications for personality disorder are not necessary unless one has signs of an illness too.

Behavior (as an action or lack of it)

Behavior is what one does. Every action we take is usually triggered by feeling and is based on thinking which leads to planning and choice. If it satisfies our needs and makes us feel good without suffering, it has a good outcome. Actions we take include: eating, drinking, making love, violence, self-intoxication, exercise, writing, painting, speaking, creating or repairing. Without these actions, there is not much of a difference between humans and plants. Actions help us to build communities or destroy them. They may help our growth and development, or hinder it. They either have a positive or negative outcome.

If the outcome of our behavior is persistently and repeatedly negative, we consider it disordered. Alcoholism, drug abuse, anorexia, sexual disorders, pathological gambling, suicide, violence and theft are examples of disordered behavior. Although they are triggered by feeling or lack of it and are planned based on thinking or lack of it, it's not the feeling and thinking that is targeted in treatment but the action itself. We can't ask someone not to feel sad or think they are worthless, but we can prevent that person from committing suicide. We cannot prevent people from having feelings of hate or prejudice, but we can help them not to act violently. We cannot convince an anorexic not to feel sad, ugly and overweight, but we can prevent the person from dying from emaciation. We cannot expect people not to feel nervous or angry and think alcohol or drugs is the answer, but we can help them to avoid engaging in intoxication, self-harm, and harming others. We cannot expect people not to have a desire for sex and think urgently that porn, rape and pedophilia is the answer, but we can prevent them from those actions and save people from getting harmed. We cannot expect an obsessed person not to worry about germs and think constantly about washing their hands, but we can help the person practice safe and monitored behaviors, such as touching dirt without washing for a while. Also, adding medications might be helpful in cases such obsessive-compulsive disorder, withdrawal from substances, or recurrent pathological sexual urges.

Life Experience

Our upbringing, education, emotions such as love, hate, violence, pleasure and joy are examples of life experiences. Specific life experiences might include losing a job or a significant other, getting married, becoming ill, traveling or winning the lottery.

Life experience has a significant impact on the way one feels, thinks and behaves. Someone who was well taken care of in life, never had the opportunity to stand on their own feet, didn't experience any hardship, and didn't have to solve any problems, might become spoiled or dependent on their significant others. If someone drives over a bridge and suddenly an earthquake causes the bridge to collapse and they witness many people die, this person will likely have a fear about driving over bridges. Experiencing traumatic events such as war or natural disasters leads to recurrent anxious feelings, helpless thinking, and avoidant behavior of any normal events that are a reminder of the trauma. These experiences frame people's behavior. The main treatment for negative framing is reframing the individual's feeling, thinking, and behavior that such events will not necessarily happen again.

The reframing of traumatic experiences gives the individual a chance to re-evaluate the negative emotion, recognize their distorted thinking and practice new behaviors. Sometimes transitional medication might help with certain symptoms such as excessive panic, sleeplessness and anxiety. Once reframing is complete, medications might no longer be necessary.

The components of perspective of psychiatry which include disease, personality, life story, and behavior are summarized in the following table.

Table of components of Psychiatric Perspective

Factor	Reason	Example
Disease	A broken part or what one has or acquired in term of medical health	Stroke, Depression, Mania, Schizophrenia, OCD, Panic etc.
Personality	A graded dimension or who one is	Intellect, height, weight, personality traits such as introversion and extroversion, shyness, suspiciousness, etc.
Life story	The narrative of what one has experience in life	Upbringing, Education, experience of love, violence, war, trauma, loss, wealth, poverty, etc.
Behavior	The action of what one does or does not do	Service or disservice to one's or society's well being such as violence, addictions, anorexia, sexual disorders, gambling etc.

Psychiatric Evaluation

Clinicians evaluate patients in a comprehensive initial interview. The interview is most helpful if the patient who is seeking help voluntarily and discloses everything, giving the clinician a better understanding and ability to develop a more accurate diagnosis and treatment plan. For those whose insight and judgment is compromised or impaired, there is no other option but to get information from those who bring the patient for help. It's also beneficial to obtain information from other colleagues who have done assessments and treatment previously. If the patient and significant others are able to give an accurate history, it might be more beneficial for a clinician to make a new comprehensive evaluation before checking with other colleagues, especially for second-opinion evaluations.

Identifying Information

The interview starts with recording the patient's demographics: age, gender, ethnicity, marital status, employment, any past mental signs and symptoms, and the main reason (in a word or so) of why the individual is seeking help. Demographics are relevant and important, as certain conditions are age-specific, such as dementia in an older person or parent–child relationship problems in teenagers. There is no need to be worried about premenstrual dysphonic disorder in a male patient or a low testosterone level in a teenage girl. Ethnicity is relevant, as there tends to be more alcohol use in Native American cultures, while there is more opiate use in the Middle East. Whether someone is in a meaningful relationship with a spouse or lover, just broke up from such a relationship, or has never had a romantic relationship makes a difference in understanding the patient. Working as a CEO, a security guard, a teacher, or being unemployed each has its own challenges for the individual seeking help. In terms of a word about past diagnosis, if one has a history of mood swings or schizophrenia, this information makes it easier to know what to look for more carefully in the evaluation. And, finally, why one is seeking help is important; whether the individual was just assaulted, has increased hallucinations, or is frustrated with excessive substance use are considered different types of chief complaints that can lead to a proper work up of the problem.

Patient's Background

After getting demographic information on the patient, typically the clinician focuses on asking about the background of the individual. This include place of birth and upbringing, growth and development, parents' profession and child-rearing style, traumatic experiences, level of education, employment, position and income, marital status, sexual orientation, having children and siblings or not, living situation, drug use, legal situation, religion or spirituality, hobbies, and strengths and weaknesses.

The background information is relevant. Growing up on in a farm or in a city may lead to different approaches to solving challenges. Whether someone has a speech impediment or delayed development, or was a very quick learner often leads to different outcome in one's life. Their parent's job and upbringing style are not all the same: some parents may live in poverty and be affectionate to their child, while others might be very wealthy yet neglectful in spending time with their children. Whether a child's parent was beaten up frequently by a neglectful, abusive and alcoholic parent has a different impact on the child's life than being raised by someone like TV's Mr. Rogers, who every morning would say "it's a beautiful day in the neighborhood".

If, as a child, the patient had difficulty at school, needed extra support they didn't receive, and/or was teased or bullied by peers, he or she would behave subsequently different from one that was a fast learner, encouraged at home, and engaged in various extracurricular activities to be more competitive in a demanding world.

Being unemployed and living in poverty differs from having a job, a nice home, plenty of food, and clothes to wear. It makes a difference if the patient is in a meaningful and loving romantic relationship, or in a constantly nagging and demeaning one, or has none of these. Having children and siblings and a relationship with them, whether caring or competitive, or whether healthy and dysfunctional, leads to a different way of coping with relationships.

The living situation of a clan family of 10 people in a small apartment is very different than the nuclear family of a couple and their two children that live in a mansion.

The person who has faced legal problems, went to jail, and had to pay a significant amount of fines may deal with minor issues differently than one who had never faced challenges with law enforcement.

The patient who has experienced mind-altering substances, abused them and has perhaps become dependent on them likely does not behave the same as one who for religious reasons never touched a substance, or the person who only occasionally has used such substances for relaxation, socialization and enjoyment. The extent, amount, consequences of using alcohol, heroin, cocaine, cannabis, tobacco and other substances helps with making the diagnosis.

Someone who is devoted to a higher idea, whether religious or humanistic or agnostic, is less likely to think that life is worthless than the person who has no spirituality and no connection to a purpose of life. The same argument can be made for having a meaningful hobby or plan to enjoy life. This background evaluation gives important insight into understanding the patient's strengths and weaknesses during therapeutic intervention.

Family History

The next step in evaluation is to learn the patient's family history. Many major illnesses might be genetic, even if they present differently in future generations. If a patient's grandfather had depression, this information can alert the doctor to look for depression, anxiety, bipolar or other major mental illnesses in the individual who is seeking help.

The family history usually refers to blood-related family members and includes information about past and present generations in the family, especially psychiatric diagnosis of parents, children and their blood relatives. This information might be helpful not only for diagnostic purposes but also for therapeutic intervention. At the same time, if a parent experienced trauma and subsequent anxiety, but was able to recover before his or her child was born, it's unlikely this has a significant impact on the diagnosis of anxiety in the child seeking help. However, the persistent worries of a parent may lead to the development of anxiety in a child.

Past Medical History

Looking into the patient's medical history is very important. Many medical conditions such as cancer, heart failure, and liver cirrhosis can have a demoralizing impact on individuals. Some medical conditions could even present with a mental disorder too. While hypothyroidism and pancreatic cancer could present with depressive syndrome, hyperthyroidism and excessive adrenalin make an individual anxious and restless. Often a laboratory work up and even imaging is necessary in an individual who presents with a new onset of psychiatric symptoms. A basic relevant physical exam, such as measuring blood pressure and heart rate and observing gait and movements, may be needed. Information about allergies, symptoms in different organ systems, relevant physical exam findings, laboratory and imaging studies, and current medications and their benefits and potential side effects belong here.

Past Psychiatric History

Gaining as much information as possible about past psychiatric history is very relevant in the initial evaluation. People might present with a depressive syndrome to a clinician. However, going beyond cross-sectional symptoms and learning about past presentations of mood changes (such as elation and euphoria) might change the suspicion about a depressive syndrome to a possible diagnosis of manic depression. The individuals past response and the response of their family members to a certain type of treatment or medication and past side effect on such makes it easier for a doctor to choose the right treatment for the patient. Information about past therapy and consultations, medications, hospitalization, rehabilitations, self-injurious behavior, and violence is also essential.

History of Present Problem

The patient usually presents with a complaint. It's important to know what the problem is and when, why, how, and for how long the problems have been going on. It's essential to look at contributing factors such as an immediate job loss, relationship problem, intoxication, traumas, medical illness, and loss of a significant other. The signs and symptoms of the individual are also very important in suspecting a diagnosis.

For example: tremors might suggest anxiety, Parkinson's disease, or intoxication by or withdrawal from certain substances. Crying and soft speech might suggest loss, depression, emotional instability and trauma. Inability to communicate and being withdrawn could be a sign of shyness, apathy, depression, or even a negative sign of psychosis. Expansive mood, evasive attitude and loud speech could be related to hypomania or mania. Being inattentive and easily distracted without other signs and

29

symptoms might be due to Attention Deficit Disorder. Memory loss, speech problem and disorientation could suggest some form of dementia.

Mental Status Examination

A mental status exam measures a person's orientation to the person, place, and date. If one does not know where or who he or she is, one could think about the possibility of dissociation, dementia, delirium, severe depression or intoxication. The level of cooperation is important, as a guarded individual might be paranoid. A person whose cooperation ranges from expansiveness to tearfulness could be going through a mixed state of a bipolar episode, or they could be exaggerating symptoms for a secondary gain. A quiet, apathetic person could be in a mute state due to loss or depression. An uncooperative person may have been forced to seek help by a significant other or by the authorities due to socially unacceptable behavior.

Observing eye contact gives a great understanding of the individual, if they are shy or aggressive. The way one walks and moves gives a good hint if one suffers from Parkinson's, familial tremor, and stimulant abuse or alcohol withdrawal.

Tone and volume of speech whether loud, soft, monotonous, organized, articulate and/or reasonable suggest some form of wellness or illness. How a patient subjectively expresses feelings whether normal, sad, nervous, happy or angry can also help the clinician understand the patient. Asking about sleep, energy, motivation, desire, concentration, appetite and/or confidence may be added to a current mental status examination. Also, whether the patient has any form of anxiety, panic, obsession, compulsion or restlessness is important in determining if they have one or another form of an anxiety disorder.

How one's thought process is expressed through speech whether concrete, articulate, organized, disorganized or nonsensical is important to determine if one is of sound mind or not. The content of thought, such as suicidal or homicidal ideation, is essential in determining if the patient's or another person's life is in an immediate danger. Asking about delusions, hallucinations, ideas of reference, thought insertion by others and/or reading other people's thoughts could be a sign of psychosis.

Whether one understands why he or she needs help, and if he/or she agrees to receive help or not, suggests the patient's level of insight and judgment.

Overall, a Mental Status Examination covers the following: cognition, orientation, movements, behavior, speech, mood, affect, desire to die passively, or suicidal and homicidal ideation, vital sign changes, changes in self-esteem, anxiety, obsession and compulsion, panic, phobia, hallucinations, delusions, general information and intelligence, insight and judgment as well as a mini -mental examination which might be more relevant in people with dementia and delirium but also in severe depression, mania, and dissociation.

Following table summarized the component of psychiatric evaluation.

Table of Components of Psychiatric Evaluation

ID	Age, gender, marital status, job, and chief compliant
Background	Place of birth, upbringing, parents position, siblings, education, profession, income, living situation, legal history, spirituality, hobbies, substance use
Family History	History of mental illness in blood related family members and treatment response
Medical History	Any medical condition past and present, laboratory and imaging studies, treatments, surgeries, physical traumas, allergies, and any current physical symptoms
Medications	Current medications
Psychiatric History	Age of first symptoms of and treatment for mental health, subsequent treatments, treatment response, hospitalization, self injurious behavior, violence
Current Psychiatric Problem	What is the problem, when did it start, how long, what are the symptoms, what are the triggers and contributing factors,
Mini Mental Status Examination	Alertness, orientation, cooperation, movements, speech, mood, affect, thought process, though content, insight and judgment

Assessment and Diagnosis

Once all the information above has been gathered, the clinician may highlight the significant and relevant factors and come up with an assessment and diagnosis. It is important to understand if the contributing factors that have led to the suffering of the patient are related to an illness, personality, a life experience, a behavior or a combination of a few or all of these. Among these factors, the clinician identifies the patient's strengths and weaknesses. The diagnosis is usually based on five axes:

Axis I includes major mental disorders such as depression, schizophrenia, bipolar, anxiety, obsessive compulsive disorder, attention deficit disorder, adjustment disorder, post traumatic disorder, alcoholism, sexual disorders, etc. Axis I includes major mental disorders such as depression, schizophrenia, bipolar, anxiety, obsessive compulsive disorder, attention deficit disorder, adjustment disorder, post traumatic disorder, alcoholism, sexual disorders, etc. This axis includes disorders that are not primarily medial or biologically based but rather based on a behavior in the case of alcoholism or a life experience in the case of post traumatic stress disorder or adjustment disorder. In my opinion, conditions such as adjustment disorder and post-traumatic stress disorder should be classified in an axis that is relevant to environmental factors, and alcoholism and sexual disorders in an axis that is behavioral. At the same time, it is understandable to leave these conditions in axis I, as they have the potential to lead to a disease due to their chronic impact on the brain and body.

Axis II includes intellectual disability and personality disorders categorized in clusters A, B, and C. Cluster A includes persons with traits such oddity, eccentric, apathy, coldness and paranoia. Cluster B people have traits such as being dramatic, self-centered, and excessively emotional. Cluster C include people with traits such as dependency on others, avoidance and obsessions. Each cluster is also subcategorized into different personality disorders. During the first and even few sessions thereafter, one cannot make a quick judgment about one's personality. In order to find out who the person is and what personality disorder they might suffer from, the patient has to be stable medically and psychiatrically. In other words a diagnosis of personality disorder can only be reasonable if the patient is free from moderate to severe medical signs and symptoms such as insomnia, loss of appetite, and suicidal thoughts to name a few. There are some suggestions that personality disorders and major mental illnesses are in a continuous spectrum. This means that cluster A people might have mild schizophrenia, while cluster B could be afflicted with milder form of bipolar illness and cluster C with milder form of anxiety and depression.

Axis III includes medical conditions that might have an impact on the psychiatric presentation of the patient who is seeking help. For example, if one has had a stroke on the left side of the brain and presents with a depressive syndrome, one could argue that the depression is due to a medical condition. Some clinicians might include all and some only the relevant medical conditions that have an impact on mental health in axis III. Ideally axis I and III should be combined into one axis and called Biological Axis.

Axis IV is about the social factors that have affected the patient negatively. Relationship problems, legal issues, educational challenges, occupational matters, cultural difficulties are some of the topics in axis IV. Ideally this axis should be named Life Experience Axis.

Axis V is for global assessment of functioning and ranges up to 100. It is unlikely for anyone to be 100% functional and have no biological, psychological and/or social problems. People who present with suicidal or homicidal urges, and those who are psychotic and do not make sense during evaluation usually have a functioning level below 40 and need close observation in a facility.

The following table is a summary of components of psychiatric diagnosis based on DSM and its correlation with perspective of psychiatry.

Table of Diagnostic Axis and Its Correlation Based On Perspective of Psychiatry

Axis	Based on DSM	Perspective	Example
I	Major mental disorder	Disease, Behavior, life story	Depression, addiction, withdrawal, PTSD, paraphilia
II	Personality and intellectual ability	Personality	Cluster A/B/C traits, Intellectual limitation, shyness, impulsivity
III	Medical conditions that contribute to mental illness	Disease	Stroke, pancreas cancer, withdrawals, CVA, autism
IV	Social and environmental factors	Life story	Education, occupation, relationship, legal issues, PTSD
V	Global assessment of function	N/A but ranges from 0 to 100	Under 45 for hospitalized patients and 90 for average person. Unlikely anyone is 100.

Treatment Plan

Upon assessment and diagnosis, the clinician comes up with a treatment plan to help the suffering individual. The plan first starts with making sure the patients are not in any immediate danger to self or others. Once this is determined, the next step is to make sure necessary medications are recommended if there is a major mental disorder. If the patient is medically and psychiatrically stable enough to participate in the learning process, different forms of psychological therapy such as cognitive behavioral therapy, dynamic therapy, supportive therapy, eclectic therapy, existential therapy or social interventions (help for education, occupation, relationships and housing) are recommended.

Major Disorders and Their Potential Treatment

Based on diagnostic classifications of mental disorders, there are hundreds of disorders. However, one can simplify them to a few. These few include: depression, bipolar disorder, schizophrenia, anxiety, personality disorders, behavioral disorders and life experience disorders.

Treatment modalities for feeling (emotion), thinking (process, content, and perception), and behavior (drive, learning) include biological (medical, genetic, neurotransmitter), psychodynamic (conflicts, interpretations), behavioral (choices, drives, motives) and biopsychosocial (eclectic, combination of approaches).

Mood Disorders

A majority of patients who seek psychiatric help have some type of mood, feeling or emotional disorder. Most of them have been diagnosed with depression. However, it is possible that most of them also have some type of cyclic mood (ups and downs). An excessive form of cyclic mood is bipolar disorder. The life of a patient who suffers from bipolar disorder might be similar to a person who lives and swims in the ocean day and night. While the person swims in a smooth ocean often, at times they could be on top of a high wave and full of energy and at times they could be exhausted and sink to the bottom of the ocean. A person in this situation needs a boat, or mood stabilizer in this analogy, in order to remain safe.

Depression

Depression is an episodic emotional or affective disorder. Episodic means that it could come and go, even without treatment. Sometimes recovery could last for months or years without proper treatment. It manifests itself in the form of sadness and diminished vitality. Depressed people lack motivation, joy, concentration, appetite and a desire for intimacy. They feel guilty or angry with themselves or others. They might see no purpose to continue living and have a desire to die or even commit suicide.

While the clinician is empathetic to the patients feeling of sadness and guilt, and even may have teary eyes when seeing that the patient is suffering, he or she tries to understand the distorted thinking of the patient and point out the flaws in such thinking. The clinician could remind the hopeless patient that despite some evidence of miseries in one's life, there is more evidence that life still offers the opportunity for recovery and improvement. If a person with renal, cardiac, and liver failure can survive and even recover via treatment, there is no reason for a patient who suffers from depression to give up hope. Just seeing a butterfly flying, a child or elderly person smiling, a river running, a flower blooming, an actor performing, a singer signing, an ill person recovering, and people helping each other in a disastrous situation are all indications that there's hope and that life is beautiful and should be cherished despite its challenges.

While showing empathy and promoting hope, the clinician's main goal is that the depressed patient avoids behavior that worsens the condition and starts actions that lead to improvement. It's important to make sure patients take eating seriously despite lack of appetite, socializing despite lack of interest, exercising despite lack of energy, reading despite lack of focus, and playing and cuddling despite lack of desire for intimacy. Another key element of therapeutic intervention is educating the significant people in the patient's life to be supportive instead of demanding. Guiding the patient to get help for lost jobs and income and to participate in a relevant support group is also very beneficial in therapy. Above all, a trial of various antidepressants is essential to make the recovery faster.

Bipolar

Like depression, bipolar illness is also an episodic emotional and affective disorder. It differs from depression in that the illness fluctuates between highs and lows or has a combination of both. Among affective disorders only depression is low. The other three main emotions such as anxiety, happiness and anger manifest in emotions that are too high. The lows of bipolar are typical depressive episodes as described above. The highs could be excessive happiness, anger or even anxiety. Some bipolar individuals might present with a few yearly episodes of mild lows and highs, this can be referred to as mood swings or cyclothymic disorder. Many individuals might function well enough without treatment for such mild changes in mood.

One could argue that everyone goes through occasional mood changes. If a patient or their significant other are bothered by such mild symptoms and would rather try medication for stability, they should have that opportunity. If the mood changes are excessive, prolonged and affect professional and interpersonal relationships, in the case of mild bipolar or Bipolar II disorder, then medical treatment is necessary. This will help reduce the patient's excessive manic symptoms such as elation, overspending, recklessness, promiscuity, anger and agitation, frequent loud arguments and fights, as well as constant anxiety, phobia and restlessness.

In the case of sever bipolar when the patient is reckless, disorganized, and incoherent, runs naked in the street, is delusional or has hallucinations, medical intervention is a must to bring the patient down to a stable and safe state of mind. Once the patient is stable via various mood stabilizers, anti-psychotics and anti-anxiety medications, other therapeutic intervention that apply to depression could be applied to mood swings, hypomania and mania as well. Since bipolar patients with hypomania and mania often make quick and risky decisions, it's important to educate them to give themselves at least 24 hours or to talk to a loved one before taking a risk. This might make the risk less dangerous or even prevent a disastrous outcome such as financial ruin or getting a sexual transmitted disease.

Anxiety

There are different forms of anxiety that include general anxiety disorder, phobias, obsessive-compulsive disorder and posttraumatic disorder (PTSD). The latter might be rather a life experience disorder, but since many people with PTSD might have had an underlying mild anxiety disorder even prior to trauma; it has been categorized as a medical condition like other forms of anxiety. I believe anxiety disorders should be placed among affective disorders like depression and mania, as it is about emotion and affect. However, anxiety disorders have their own category in the DSM.

General anxiety disorder presents with constant worries about many things ranging from what shirt to wear to future survival. The patient is restless and cannot sleep well due to excessive worries, and often anticipates that something could go wrong.

In the case of obsessive-compulsive disorder, the anxious feeling is more specific and the individual engages in a repetitive behavior to neutralize recurrent obsessive thoughts. One might feel dirty and worry about germs and wash his or her hands repeatedly. One might be worried about a break-in and check the doors and windows multiple times. The patient might be concerned about fire and check the stove over and over. Or they may be worried about something unusual happening if they do not do certain actions in a specific way, such as avoiding cracks on a pathway. Often there are a certain number of repetitive actions that OCD patients have to take before they can rest. In contrast to delusional patients, people who suffer from OCD are aware that their behavior does not make sense, yet they cannot control it.

Some anxious people suffer from phobia and it could range from germs to people, closed places, flying on airplanes or driving a car. They might have had a bad experience or heard about one and have an underlying nervousness that leads them to avoid the setting or situation.

In people who have witnessed a trauma and developed PTSD, they may become hyper-vigilant, easily startled, sleepless, and angry, have flashbacks and avoid any situation that reminds them of the trauma.

People who have panic disorder often present with certain physiological symptoms that are perceived as life threatening by the patients. These symptoms include increased hearth rate, shortness of breath, nausea, diarrhea, tingling and chest pain.

Most antidepressants are beneficial in the treatment of all anxiety disorders. In fact, one might consider antidepressants emotional regulators. However, they should not be confused with mood stabilizers, which reduce mania and hypomania. In addition to antidepressants, mood stabilizers and antipsychotics may reduce the level of anxiety and obsessive preoccupations. Unless the patient suffers from other major illness that leads to suicidal or homicidal thoughts, anxious patients can usually be treated in an outpatient setting and hospitalization will most likely not be needed. For temporary relief of some symptoms of anxiety and panic, one might also use benzodiazepines. This category of anti-anxiety medications tends to cause dependency and is usually avoided by clinicians. However, some patients might need to be on medications forever to live a normal life.

Thought Disorders

Thought disorders include conditions in which the patient's thinking process or content or both is not normal. It could range from severe conditions such as schizophrenia and dementia to a less troubling condition such as inattention.

Schizophrenia

Schizophrenia is one of the most serious mental illnesses. In contrast to episodic affective disorder, schizophrenia is usually a steady thought disorder. Once one is afflicted with this illness, return to a pre-morbid condition is unlikely. However, to be hopeful, there is always treatment that prevents worsening and even makes the patient function at some level. As an example a professor who was recently diagnosed with schizophrenia could not likely continue to function as a professor in academia due to the severity of his condition; however he may be able to do a less demanding task appropriate for his compromised ability. In the beginning of biological psychiatry, schizophrenia was called dementia praecox, as patients with this affliction lost the capacity of their thinking at an early age, just as an elderly patient with Alzheimer's would. Different types of schizophrenia, such as paranoid, disorganized, catatonic and undifferentiated, were considered at some point. Now the tendency is to consider all types as one illness with different presentations.

The symptoms of schizophrenia may include disorganized behavior and speech, delusions, hallucinations and apathy. The reality of a patient who has schizophrenia is different than the one of non-psychotic people, as they cannot be convinced that their fixed false thoughts about reality are not real. Because of the severity of their compromised thinking capacity and functioning, they might have a better chance of a comfortable life in a less stimulating setting such as a rural area than a high demanding metropolis. In the pre-enlightenment era, these patients might have been chained in a cellar by their family or by the government. Fortunately, we now have treatment options that reduce the suffering of these patients so they may be able to have a decent life whether it's in a state facility, board and care housing, or among understanding family members. With treatment, patients with schizophrenia gradually become used to the hallucinations and delusions they might still have. While they might remain suspicious and eccentric, they can interact with others who understand them. Conventional psychotherapy without medications is probably useless for such patients, as they might not trust others easily or lack the interest or capacity to participate in such therapies. However, anti-psychotics have done wonders in terms of reducing symptoms and improving the lives of many patients with schizophrenia.

Other Psychotic Disorders

Schizoaffective disorder is when an individual suffers from the illness that has the symptoms of both schizophrenia and affective or mood disorder. It might not be as severe as schizophrenia and the affective part of it could be episodic. This means that depression, mania or hypomania of people with schizoaffective disorder may resolve yet psychotic symptoms such as delusions and hallucinations may persist. Another related condition is affective disorder with psychotic features. In contrast to schizoaffective disorder, individuals with affective disorder that have a psychotic component will have resolution of the psychotic symptoms when the affective disorder resolves. Other psychotic disorders include single delusional disorder which is characterized by paranoia without hallucinations. Usually any psychotic disorder without a prior disorder is called Psychosis NOS. Schizophrenia is a diagnosis of exclusion and is diagnosed after six months of observation to rule out other psychotic disorders.

Attention Deficit Disorder

Attention-deficit/hyperactivity disorder (ADHD) could be considered primarily a thought disorder. It is about the inability to focus, forgetfulness, distractibility, fidgetiness, hyperactivity and impulsivity. However, these symptoms are related to the frontal part of the brain rather than the emotional part, and therefore these clusters of symptoms are related to thinking and executive functioning. Unlike patients with a serious thought disorder such as schizophrenia, patients with attention deficit disorder might enjoy a fruitful life even without treatment. In addition to cognitive behavioral therapy to avoid impulsivity, medications could help with inattention and hyperactivity. While stimulants that are similar to amphetamine are beneficial, there is a risk of abuse and dependency. Other non-stimulant medications such as bupropion or atomaxatine maybe as beneficial as stimulants and have no risk of abuse or dependency.

Dementia

Different types of dementia also lead to distorted thought processes, and impairments in memory and executive functioning. Recovery to baseline functioning in dementia is not possible. Educating the family and assuring the patients safety is the key in treatment. Various medications are also used to slow down the progress of dementia. Since dementia is primarily a neurological disorder, we leave it to our neurology colleagues who are experts in these conditions to further explain and treat these conditions.

Behavioral Disorders

Behavior is something that one does and not what one is, has, or experienced. Like religion and sexuality that are private matters, it is no one's business to tell any adult with normal intelligence how to behave unless the behavior is hurting somebody. In the case of some behavioral disorders, it's usually the misbehaving person who is suffering most. In other cases, innocent people might get hurt and so the intensity of the intervention differs from one disorder to the other.

Why should one bother a chain smoker whose pleasure is to have as many puffs as he or she wants, unless the individual decides to increase his or her chance of a longer life span and prevent a potential lung cancer?

It is no one's business to tell a paraphiliac person who is addicted to porn or has pleasure with some else's foot what to do. Yet, if this person is overwhelmed with his or her behavior and spends hours acting on the urges, loses a job and a spouse, and asks for help, then the person should receive proper care without judgment.

A similar egalitarian argument could be made for people with anorexia, bulimia, and body dysmorphic disorders who go through multiple surgeries. As long as they remain functional and hurt no one, why should one not let them do what they think makes them happy. But again, some anorexics might lose so much weight that it results in death, and bulimics might be so dehydrated that could have a seizure, hit their head and die, and body dysmorphic disordered people could remain disappointed for not achieving their goal ever and kill themselves. In such cases and to save lives, treatment is essential.

There are cases of various behavioral disorders such as recurrent and excessive abuse of cannabis, alcohol, heroin, cocaine and prescription drug abuse. If an individual becomes dependent and intoxicated on such substances or goes through withdrawal, which may become a life threatening medical condition, it causes a loss of capacity to think clearly. These individuals may make poor decisions, drive while disoriented, and get in an accident and put themselves and others in danger. In such cases, the treatment is usually imposed by the court.

In a severe case of behavioral disorder such as pedophilia it is not the individual who is suffering primarily but an innocent person who does not have the capacity to make a decision and is being taken advantage of by an offender. For such a case, judgment and punishment is justified unless the offender himself or herself is very ill mentally and has no capacity to make the right choice. Regardless of the capacity, treatment is mandatory in such a case.

The main treatment for all behavioral disorders, which are mainly acted out in secret, is to be honest about their existence and stop or change them to an acceptable behavior. One's setting often needs to be changed in order for the behavior to stop. An alcoholic or drug abuser should avoid any setting where there is a temptation to relapse. A patient with anorexia or bulimia needs to be open about the urges and not be left alone, even in the bathroom, and should be accompanied by a loved one to prevent relapse until the maladaptive behavior has become extinct. The same reassuring and supportive control could be done for someone with paraphilia. In the case of a pedophile, it is not safe for him or her to work at a setting where there is exposure to minors.

While different forms of psychotherapy are beneficial for behavioral disorders, the key again is stopping the behavior and removing the individual from a tempting setting. In addition to psychotherapy and controlling the behavior to stop, some medications might be necessary to make the transition to an acceptable lifestyle possible. For example, benzodiazepines might be helpful to prevent withdrawal from alcohol, and a prescribed opiate might be necessary to reduce the pain of heroin addicts. Antidepressants, mood stabilizers and antipsychotics could also be helpful as transitional tool to help the patient stop their unhealthy behavior. There are also some medications such as opiate antagonists that might reduce the urges of bulimics, alcoholics and opiate abusers. Probably the most effective therapy for people with behavioral disorders is anonymous group therapy.

Personality Clusters

As mentioned before, personality disorders are grouped in A, B and C clusters. Cluster A include paranoid, schizoid, and schizotyipal personality disorders. Cluster B includes histrionic, narcissistic, borderline and antisocial personality disorders. Cluster C include obsessive-compulsive personality, dependent, and avoidant and, for some, maybe depressive personality disorders. While cluster A might be in the spectrum of schizophrenia, cluster B resembles some form of bipolarity, and cluster C maybe milder forms of anxiety and depressive disorder.

The features of cluster A might include oddity, eccentricity, suspiciousness, apathy or lack of interest in various subjects, withdrawal from society, being superstitious, preoccupied with conspiracy thoughts, etc. In contrast to patients with schizophrenia, these patients do not have hallucinations and delusions. Some great scientists might be among them and in their isolative world make a great contribution to the society. While the ideas of patients with schizophrenia are fixed and false and therefore delusional, the ideas of patients with cluster A personality disorder might be overvalued ideas with a possibility of some truth to them. These patients might even be able to doubt that their ideas could be false.

Supportive and understanding therapy is probably the best choice for these patients. Since they don't trust others easily or their thinking style differs from average people, it is unlikely they would benefit from group therapy. If they present with transitional additional symptoms of anxiety, depression and psychosis, medications might be helpful. If those symptoms persist, diagnosis could be modified.

Cluster B personality disorder people could be too emotional or dramatic, sensitive, self-centered; they might seek attention and desire admiration and praise, and think they are more important than others. In severe cases of people with antisocial personality disorder, they might even engage in misconduct and violate other person's right so that they can serve themselves. Despite their self-centered attitude, they have the capacity to care about their loved ones. Even dictators throughout history most likely loved their significant others. While artists, actors, and singers might have minor harmless traits of cluster B and flourish by people admiring their artistic ability, dictators have more traits of antisocial personality disorder or psychopathy. It is probably for that reason that they are merciless in violating other people and easily order killings, massacres and genocide.

Treatment of people with cluster B traits is regulation of emotions, educating them that people are created equal and deserve the same rights and attention. It's teaching them that being humble might be more effective to get where they want to be, and that life is not only about taking but also giving. In severe cases of patients with psychopathic disorder, it's essential that they are redirected from urges to violate other people's rights and they must be stopped from harming anyone. In some cases, these people might present with symptoms of emotional disorder that requires either transitional or continuous medication. Dialectical behavioral therapy (DBT) might also be a better option for these individuals compared to other forms of psychotherapy.

The Cluster C personality disorder group may be dependent, indecisive without reassurance by others, clingy, perfectionistic, moralistic, rigid, and careful with money, shy, withdrawn and may be depressed. The three defined categories include avoidant, dependent and obsessive-compulsive personality disorders. They might be in the spectrum of mood or affective disorder. However, the symptoms are not as severe as to be considered medical condition such as anxiety and depression.

Any form of therapy would be helpful in terms of helping individuals to practice socialization, rely on themselves and not be overwhelmed by criticism. In terms of a job, they might be somewhat perfectionist and reliable and, considering their characteristics, might fit in a position with limited social interaction. They might do a better job as accountant, librarians and laboratory scientists or workers.

If they develop symptoms of anxiety, depression and obsession, they would benefit from medication.

Life Experience Disorders

We all face various life challenges from childhood until the end of our lives. Being neglected or abused versus being loved and taken care of by every means would have a different outcome on how we behave. Depending on other factors such as education, emotional and financial support later in life, things could turn around. It's not guaranteed that love and support would necessarily turn someone into a loving and productive individual. If the individual's underlying predisposition is towards anger and acting out, even the most loved person might turn out to be the opposite of what his or her parents expect. Someone who had a very rough childhood might have become very self-reliant and, in turn, live a productive life. Often parents blame themselves for bad outcomes and ignore various factors in their children's life. It is ultimately the parent's responsibility to do their best and if something goes wrong, adapt and change their parenting style. Not only during childhood but throughout life, we are exposed to challenges that impact our lives.

Adjustment Disorder

If one has been fired or lost significant others, it's normal to be sad and disappointed. Usually people eventually adjust to such losses. However, if sadness persists beyond what is average and the patient develops signs and symptoms of depression and anxiety and has no other identifiable factors but the loss, then adjustment disorder would be the right diagnosis. In case of the loss of significant others, bereavement would be a more appropriate name for the condition. If the level of depression and anxiety are too excessive and persist for too long, one might consider treating them with medications in addition to psychotherapy. Otherwise, attending support group would be helpful.

Demoralization

Sufferings from any serious medical condition such as cancer or HIV, for which treatment is limited, would be demoralizing for anyone. Like other forms of adjustment disorder, the same treatment can apply to demoralization.

Post-Traumatic Stress Disorder

Anyone who has witnessed a life-threatening event would most likely go through anxiety and restlessness, have nightmares, be easily startled and become depressed and angry. Post Traumatic Stress Disorder (PTSD) was named when many veterans reported such symptoms after they had returned from the Vietnam War. Not only war but also other tragic experiences such as sexual assault, a car crash, or an earthquake could lead to PTSD. If someone witnessed an earthquake while driving over a bridge, it is unlikely that he or she would be able to drive over another bridge without proper treatment. PTSD and bridge phobia might be the outcome of such an experience. There are arguments that people with a milder form of pre-morbid anxiety are at a higher risk for developing PTSD.

Empathy, support, reassurance and reframing of distorted thoughts that one does not have to relive these traumatic experiences again are the cornerstone of therapy. Group therapy under the supervision of a therapist and with people who have similar experiences is also of significant benefit. Medications might be necessary to help with persistent anxiety, anger and depression.

Medications

As stated earlier, the role of medication in the brain could be compared to the role of oil in a factory that functions by many interconnected wheels. To continue to function without breakdown, the wheels have to be oiled on a regular basis. The factory has the oil in it, but it might leak or flow slowly or too rapidly. Similarly, the brain has the neurotransmitters within itself, but it might be insufficient in a place where it is supposed to be.

The choice of medications depends on various factors such as prior response, response of a biologically related family member, symptoms, and side effect potential. Since the development of modern and effective medications such as lithium, tricyclic antidepressants and typical antipsychotics in the middle of 20th century, many new medications with fewer side effects have come to the market. Usually if the person has not had any prior experience with the medications, the clinician tries to choose the safest or mildest and most cost-effective one.

Some patients argue that they "don't believe in medications", as if medications represent a faith. They think medications are pushed by pharmaceutical companies to make a profit. This argument is flawed in several ways. Of course pharmaceutical companies want to make a profit, but their products have rescued millions of lives. It is similar to saying I "don't believe in cars" and I'd rather take a natural method for transportation, such as a bike or a horse. The fact is that most of the time the risk of medications is less than their benefit. By contrast, the risk of natural remedies could prolong the journey to recovery.

Antidepressants

Antidepressants include older tricyclics, SSRIs, MAOIs and novel agents. Tricyclic antidepressants such as nortriptyline, amitriptyline and anfranil are very effective in moderate to severe depression and anxiety. However, they have more potential side effects such as weight gain and constipation; and in overdose they could lead to heart block. So, typically, other safer agents are first tried unless they don't work. SSRIs such as fluoxetine, paroxetine, sertraline, citalopram and escitalopram are used more often, which are safer in case of overdose. Mono-Amine Oxidase Inhibitors (MAOI) are also used if SSRI and tricyclic antidepressants do not help the patient. However, MAOIs are not often the first choice, as a special diet is needed. Food that could increase the level of Mono-Amines, such as fava beans, certain cheeses and wine, should be avoided. If a patient has been on tricyclics and SSRIs, MAOIs medications can't be started without a two-week washout period to prevent drug-drug interaction. Novel agents such as venlafaxine, bupropion, mirtazapine and duloxetine can also be used and are safer than tricyclics and MAOIs. If an adequate dosage of one antidepressant is only partially helpful, a second antidepressant may be added. Sometimes other medications could be added to augment the effect of antidepressants; these augmenting agents include medications such as thyroid, lithium, estrogen, antipsychotics and stimulants.

Anti-manic Medications

Various anti-manic agents can be tried for different forms of bipolar from the mildest mood swing-cyclothymia- to Bipolar I with more severe mania. Lithium was the first effective medication for bipolar and is still among the best for severe bipolar disorder. It has a few side effects such as weight gain, tremor, kidney, and thyroid side effects, and can be toxic in the case of an overdose. Many anti-seizure medications such as valproic acid, carbamazepine and lamotrigine are also very effective in treatment of bipolar disorder. The first two could have potential side effects such as reduced platelet count and increased liver enzymes in the liver, and therefore blood monitoring is necessary. Lamotrigine is easier to manage and helps with depression in addition to mania, but it might cause a rash, which could be serious in some cases. Neuroleptic or antipsychotic medications are another choice for bipolar disorder. They not only help with severe condition such as psychosis, but they help with mania, mood swings and anxiety, and can be augmented as antidepressants.

Anti-psychotic Medications

These groups of medications are also called neuroleptics. They are categorized in two groups: typical and atypical. Typical are older and can be high or low potency and atypical are relatively newer in the market. High potency typical antipsychotics such as haloperidol and fluphenazine have more side effects such as movement disorders and in severe case narcoleptic malignant syndrome that could be life threatening. Low potency medications such as thioridazines are less likely to cause movement disorder, but may cause more weight gain. The first atypical antipsychotic was clozapine, which is helpful for people who didn't benefit from older antipsychotic medications. However, the risk of reduced white blood cell count makes it less desirable to use; blood needs to be monitored closely. Other atypical antipsychotics include quetiapine, olanzapine, risperidone, aripiprazole and ziprasidone. This group's potential side effect includes high fat level, diabetes and weight gain.

Anti-anxiety Medications

Most antidepressants and antipsychotic medications are also helpful for anxiety disorders. For panic disorder and other anxiety disorders, benzodiazepines such as lorazepam, alprazolam and clonazepam may be used. They are faster in treating panic and anxiety. However, anything quick is less reliable than anything that takes time to work. Benzodiazepine has the potential for abuse and dependency, especially in people who have a history of substance abuse. Therefore, it's not strongly recommended unless the patient isn't responding to other medications. These groups of medications are the treatment of choice for those who are dependent on any benzodiazepine or alcohol and plan to stop their dependency. A tapering-down regimen of these medications is necessary to prevent withdrawal symptoms such as elevated blood pressure and seizure.

ADHD Medications

Attention deficit hyperactive disorder is a condition that usually starts in childhood. It was thought that it resolves by adulthood. However, many adults ranging from college students to sales people and CEOs complain of a lack of attention, distractibility, and poor time management. Unless a person has a secretary to organize their schedule and help with assignments, medication could be beneficial. Stimulants such as amphetamine and methylphenidate are helpful in the treatment of ADHD. Because of their abuse and dependency potential they are not ideal. Medications such as Bupropion (an antidepressant) and atomoxatine (initially made for anxiety) are probably better choices for people with ADHD who have a history of abuse of medications.

Medications for Behavioral Preventions

Some medications are helpful in preventing relapse in recurrent addictive behavior. This includes naltrexone to reduce cravings for purging, alcoholism and opiate use; lisdexamfetamine to prevent binging; and bupropion and varenicline to stop smoking.

Procedural Therapies

Although it might have a bad reputation, electroconvulsive therapy is one of the best treatments for severe depression that is treatment refractory to medications or those who cannot take medications in the case of pregnant women with severe depression. A close analogy to ECT is cardioversion for individuals whose heart stops beating. With severe depression, the neuronal firing of the brain has been compromised significantly to a point similar to cardiac arrest. A trial of shock treatments has the potential to bring the brain back to a state of proper neuronal firing. This procedure is done under the supervision of a psychiatrist and anesthesiologist, as well as nursing staff. One of the main concerns is loss of memory for a few months; otherwise it is a very safe procedure.

Electromagnetic stimulation is similar to ECT. It might not be as effective as ECT yet this option is available for people with mild depression who are reluctant to take medications.

Vagus Nerve stimulation is showing some promise in some neurological disorders and might become the treatment of choice for depression.

Therapy Modalities

Conventional dynamic therapy was the main style of treatment for mental disorders for decades prior to other therapies or medications. In addition to various forms of dynamic therapy, other therapeutic modalities such as hypnotic, cognitive behavioral, biologically informed, dialect behavioral, supportive, family, existential, eclectic and group therapy are used by clinicians based on their training, expertise and experience.

Dynamic Therapy

Dynamic or "Freudian" therapy is based on the impact of childhood experiences that lead to different levels of moral development, value systems and conflict resolution. Although Freud might not have been a master of conventional morality, he thought that the id, ego, and superego are stages of moral development. One who is at the id stage remains self-centered and satisfies his or her needs as an adult the way a child was satisfying them when hungry or thirsty. A person at the ego stage may be in better control of satisfying his or her needs, due to fear from higher authorities such as parents, government or God. At the superego stage, one's attitude, behavior and value system is at a more mature level of development. If a self-actualized person does not act unethically, it's not due to fear but because of a developed value system.

In dynamic therapy, the clinician tries to discover life experiences such as neglect, abuse, unfulfilled wishes, lack of love and attention or competition for such. These experiences affect the child's personality, behavior and conflict resolution during his or her life span. He or she might unconsciously perceive the attitude of an employer or a therapist as similar to what he or she experienced from one of his or her parents. This concept is called transference. Another example is with the assessment of an Oedipus complex in a patient who might have been in competition with his father for the love of his mother. Dynamic therapy takes too long and might be unaffordable for many patients. A new version of it, short-term dynamic psychotherapy, might be quicker and more affordable. In this modality, the clinician identifies the underlying conflict of the patient during the therapeutic process and leads him or her to go through intensive expression and imaginary revenge in the case of a past painful experience by an offender. In his or her imagination the patient might kill the offender, go through catharsis and relief, and be pleased that the killing was only imaginary.

Cognitive Behavioral Therapy

Cognitive behavioral therapy (CBT) is about the understanding of behavior patterns and changes that one needs to make in order to change problems in the here and now. In this modality, the clinician identifies distorted thoughts and challenges them, encouraging the individual to modify them or choose an alternative behavior or way of coping with life challenges. For example, a person may feel sad and think he or she is worthless and that there is no hope for the future and the world. In this case, the clinician challenges the individual's negative beliefs and helps her or him see the positive aspects of their achievements, various beauties in the world, and see the progress from the past to the present to realize that there is hope for the future. If a patient has experienced assault and pain, the clinician might encourage him or her to consider the offender as an animal with a limited capacity to understand other people rights. It is easier to forgive an animal than a person who on a superficial level comes across as normal, yet acts inhumane and violent when he or she has a chance to hurt others in service of himself or herself.

Dialectical Behavioral Therapy

A modified version of CBT is dialectical behavioral therapy. It is ideal for the patients who have poorly-regulated emotions and behavioral urges to harm themselves. The goal is to increase their mindfulness and tolerance to stressful situations, and use positive and productive behavior to cope with them. As an example if one plans to turn an emotional pain into a physical pain by cutting her or his wrist, the DBT therapist gives the patient the tools to use a different strategy in such a situation such as going for a hike or screaming as loud as possible on top of a hill.

Hypnotherapy

Hypnotherapy is used to discover memories that have been forgotten from consciousness, yet have a significant impact on the patient's life. It is done while the patient is awake yet in a hypnotic, sleep-like state.

Supportive Therapy

Supportive therapy is about empathic listening, understanding the patient's concerns, and giving hope and encouragement that things will be better. Imagine the patient is in the middle of the ocean and does not know where to go. The fact that someone is there and can throw a rope to bring the patient to the shore is reassuring.

Group Therapy

Group therapy can be done with or without the presence of clinicians, primarily for treatment of behavioral disorders.

Alcoholics Anonymous (AA) is usually done by people who have acknowledged their addiction to alcohol, share their history and coping styles with their peers, and try to remain abstinent by attending routine meetings. Anonymous group therapy is also available for eating disorders, substance abuse, sexual disorders, gambling and more. National Alliance on Mental Illness (NAMI) offers meetings and support groups in various cities and states for people with chronic mental illness and their families.

Biologically Informed Therapy

Biologically informed therapy educates the patient about how biology and brain chemistry cause major mental disorders, and educates patients about the benefit of biological and therapeutic intervention in recovery. It helps with overcoming the stigma about mental illness and understanding that biological interventions are beneficial and quick in treating various mental disorders.

Family Therapy

Family therapy is done when, during therapy, the clinician identifies patterns of miscommunication and dysfunction in the family. It might include education about the patient's condition and the need for understanding by other family members. It can also be extensive and have many family members participate in treatment and learn to modify their own coping style with challenges at home. While at times frequent family gatherings and open communication might be needed, at other times, allowing a break from one each other might be the treatment of choice. The purpose of family therapy is to resolve a conflict in one way or the other. Imagine both sides of a conflict are as rigid as a brick. If one holds a brick in each hand and claps, the likelihood that both bricks break is high. On the other hand, if one holds a brick in one hand and a soft rubber ball in the other, clapping the hands won't cause a break. The flexibility of the ball prevents the breakage. Imagine both hand hold a soft ball. The clapping leads to bouncing. The goal is to help at least one of the conflicting parties reach a level of flexibility that can bounce in case of a disagreement. If both sides reach such a level of flexibility, the relationship might be bouncing and playful. This concept of promoting flexibility and understanding could apply to other forms of conflict resolutions between various parties.

Existential Therapy

Existential therapy is based on the philosophical understanding of one's existence and life challenges. In this method of therapy, the clinician tries to understand the ultimate fear of the patient, death. Death is inevitable and the goal is to accept it despite unfulfilled wishes. If one counts into consideration that based on his or background and resources one has accomplished all he or she could, then a natural death is nothing to worry about. The other aspect of existential theory is freedom. Understanding that freedom can only exist with its inherent responsibility could help the patient process his or ambivalence about what it means to be free. If one cannot process this ambivalence, the next step is to avoid triggers and remove or isolate oneself from life stressors that cause the ambivalence. At that stage one might come to the conclusion that the meanings and meaninglessness differ for different people and so one can live with existing realities and variations.

Eclectic Therapy

Eclectic therapy is using various therapeutic modalities based on an understanding of the patient's concerns and challenges. Depending on what the patient is going through, the therapy could range from supportive reassurance for the here and now to a deeper understanding about childhood conflicts and philosophical questions about one's existence and the meaning of life.

Examples of Practice Challenges

While a comprehensive evaluation (biological, psychological, and social) of the patient applies to everyone who seeks psychiatric help, every patient has a unique life, and unique strengths and weakness, and therefore requires an individualized assessment and treatment plan. The assessment and plan might be limited by stigma, the patient's and/or patient's family's view on mental health, their insurance plan, and the experience of the clinician.

Stigma and Fear of Medications

Often people with mental illness avoid seeking help due to the stigma of being called "crazy". Undoubtedly there is still stigma about mental illness, and more so in less-developed societies and communities. Even when someone seeks help, at times the person or the family might not be willing to try medication not only due to the fear of dependency and side effects, but also the fear of judgment by others.

I had a teenage patient accompanied by his mother. He had moderate to severe depression with intermittent suicidal thoughts. Upon a comprehensive assessment, I recommended that the sooner they start with an antidepressant, the quicker recovery would begin. The mother was very unhappy with my judgment and questioned how I could make such a recommendation after only one visit. While the patient understood my concern and was ready to accept any form of treatment, the unsatisfied mother decided to leave without further discussion. To make sure the patient receives treatment somehow, the mother agreed to take her son to another clinician for a second opinion.

Level of Care and Insurance

Treatment for mental disorders used to be available only for those who could afford it. Now due to the availability of insurances, many people can see a clinician for the challenges of their mind. At times it's difficult to convince insurance companies to cover certain treatments because of cost or effectiveness of care. They might limit the number of sessions needed for complete recovery. At times they might be concerned about the patient's safety without knowing the patient, so cooperation between the clinician and insurance company is important to make sure the patient receives proper care.

A patient of mine, who had been under my care for over a decade for episodic symptoms and had been hospitalized a few times, had recurrent suicidal thoughts in an episode. I suggested hospitalization to the patient and her family. They were reluctant and argued that previous hospitalization had not made much of a difference. Once the patient and her family agreed drafted a contract that the patient will be safe and not hurt herself, I suggested a less intensive care treatment, such as a day treatment program which would allow the patient to go home and be with her family at night so that she could relearn her forgotten coping skills and learn new ones. The case manager of her insurance refused the suggested treatment and insisted that she needs to go to a hospital due to her suicidal thoughts. We bypassed their insistence and sent the patient to the day program and instructed the patient and the family what to do meanwhile when at home. We agreed that if she cannot do anything else, she could at least watch movies with a powerful message about mental illness and hope such as "Silver Lining's Playbook". The plan was fruitful and within a week of being in the day program, the patient's suicidal urges subsided without having to go to the hospital. Subsequently, the insurance company was notified about the patient's progress without hospitalization and approved payment to the day program, which had originally been refused.

Complaint to Insurance

In the middle of the night a patient with chronic suicidal thoughts called to say that those thoughts had increased. I suggested that if the thoughts could not be controlled until a visit the next day, he should go to the emergency room. He did not like that suggestion and hung up the phone and would not answer it.

I notified 911 to go to the patient's home and evaluate the situation. He had left home upon seeing the ambulance. Later he filed an angry complaint to his insurance about being humiliated in his neighborhood by the doctor who had sent an ambulance. My response was that at baseline the patient is a gentle soul and that neither his increased suicidal thoughts nor his anger at me were typical despite a chronic negative view about life. The patient left my practice and the case was closed. After one year the patient returned to my care with an apology and I welcomed his return.

Artistic Expression

I had a very unique experience in a case of a remarkable artist with bipolar disorder. The patient was not able to express herself verbally but had the option of seeing me as needed. She could not afford frequent visits, but her insurance gave her unlimited access to care. Upon detecting the patient's artistic capability, I encouraged painting images and writing poetry. It took a series of dark images and follow-ups almost daily for the patient to write a poem reflective of mood changes and recovery. The patient recovered within two months, started communicating openly, needed less follow ups and brought images of beauties in life to discuss.

Imaginary Violence

Erroneously violence is often attributed to mental illness, while statistically patients with mental disorders are less likely to be violent than the general population. It's important to educate the public that mental illness can happen to anyone regardless of age, gender, sex, ethnicity and background. Anyone who seeks help for challenges of the mind should receive the same sympathy, empathy and respect that an individual is seeking help for any medical condition. There's also a general assumption among some lay people that imaginary violence could lead to acting violently. However, most clinicians believe imagining violence reduces the chance of acting it out.

One of my patients had been severely traumatized by an abusive spouse and developed anxiety and posttraumatic stress disorder. After targeting some physiological symptoms such as sleeplessness and anxiety, the patient was advised about short-term imaginary and expressive therapy. We tried a course of short-term dynamic therapy. The patient was led to imagine being powerful and having no inhibitions, and soon started imaginary revenge. In that visit, she imagined her spouse was tied up, dragged behind a car, driven for a while, cut in pieces and burned. Once there was no remaining trace of the spouse, the patient felt relieved and was glad her revenge was only in her imagination.

Dream

A patient had a bothersome dream and wanted to know its meaning. Dreams seem to be a combination of various experiences by our five senses. The experiences may have happened, or the person might have seen, heard or read about them. Imagine these experiences are sheets of paper put on top of each other chronologically. The order makes sense if one goes page by page from the beginning to the end. Now imagine that 10 pages are blown away by the wind and gathered again out of order. That is what a dream is like.

The patient had dreamed that she was pregnant in the labor ward and no one was there. She felt the baby's arms coming out. Her mother told her pull it out and cut the cord, but afterwards the patient didn't know what happened to the baby. She didn't know what to make of her dreams. I suggested a review of her condition and we did: She was in the process of moving to a new city to continue her education; she had a close relationship with her mother and was dependent on her support and advice; she was not sure what would happen to her in her education and career. Gradually she recognized that cutting the cord in the dream might mean that she is becoming independent from her mother, and that she is starting a new challenge in her life that is anxiety provoking.

By discussing her dream, the patient had an "aha" experience. The components of the dream included the patient's knowledge about the birth and cord, her mother as her support system, the unknown future of the baby and college student. These were different pages of a stack of papers in the patient's memory files.

Now, one could argue that the brain tries to file the patient's anxiety about moving to a new city and going to college. During a dream, the brain is searching for a category of similar stresses and finds the closest match, which in this was case the birth of a baby.

Delirium versus Dementia

I sent one of my elderly patients to a hospital for worsening depressive symptoms and confusion due to possible delirium. Unfortunately neither the admitting doctor nor I had the chance to initiate a discussion about the case. In the hospital, the patient was diagnosed with dementia and depression based on feelings of sadness, confusion, forgetfulness and fear. Luckily another medical colleague noted a urinary tract infection in the patient's laboratory work and treated the infection. The patient then was released with the residual depressive symptoms, but carried the diagnosis of dementia. Upon the first follow up visit after being discharged from the hospital, the patient could not have been happier once they were informed that the diagnosis of dementia had been made in error. The delirium had resolved and the diagnosis of dementia should have been removed upon discharge. However, imposed short stays in the hospital might be a reason that diagnoses in such a setting are not cleared before discharge.

A Couple's Relationship

A couple consulted me for the challenges in their relationship. They considered themselves as polyamorous and were about to try new relationships while keeping the unit of the family. They argued that life is short, being in various romantic relationships is not a sin, and no one has returned to give us the truth about an afterlife. The argument that smelling only one flower, eating only one fruit, and traveling only to one place is not what adult life is about seemed reasonable. The fact that great thinkers such as Simone de Beauvoir and Jean-Paul Sartre had a similar relationship, made it plausible that many other people could do the same, if that's what makes them content and happy.

The couple started their new lifestyle. After a few trials of new experiences, the couple could no longer go on. Jealousy developed and the family unit was broken. While one of them had a sense of liberation, the other was going through the pain of jealousy, loss and anger. My ultimate recommendation was that, as clinicians, we are not here to judge and solve problems, but to help patients make a choice and accept the consequences.

Special Cases

The following cases are special. Evaluation in Absentee is a hypothetical case. Mood and creativity is an interest of mine. Finally the case of chronic vomiting and related literature review is a reminder to the students and residents that they may contribute to our field not only be helping patients but by documenting and sharing interesting cases.

Evaluation in Absentee, The Case of Mr. Q

It's not unusual for friends and family members to ask questions about the mental health of a significant other. The general rule is that clinicians should not diagnose anyone without the patient being present and evaluated. However, we might be asked questions about the mental health of someone and give our opinion, if the individual remains anonymous. The following case is a typical example of evaluation in absentee. It is a formulated opinion based on presented information.

According to the inquirer, Mr. Q was an indigenous tribal leader who had died in his sixties many years ago. The inquirer was curious about the reason for his mood changes and what one should do if a descendant should go through similar changes.

When Mr. Q was born, he was considered an orphan, as his father had died before his birth. Because of the tribal tradition, he was raised by his grandfather who himself died two years later. He then returned to his mother around age five and she soon died too. Subsequently one of his uncles, a prominent and influential tribe leader, took care of him until he married. His romantic life started in his late teens when he fell in love and married a wealthy and influential widow twice as old as him. They had two sons and four daughters. Both of his sons died at a very young age. Soon the wife passed away too, after which he had become depressed and reluctant to marry again. Eventually he overcompensated and married many times including some very young girls. He had no history of alcohol and drug use. His career started with working as a farmer during his

73

teens. Soon he accompanied his uncle on trading trips and became a skillful tradesman. He was righteous and developed hostility against the elite which in his view were corrupt. He had refused an offer to join the elite, and become a warrior instead. By his late fifties he had become a renowned warrior and had won many fights. He established himself as a powerful fighter, yet had a constant worry about his rivals.

According to his friends he had been a clever, trustworthy, faithful, courageous, righteous, strong and successful fighter in the tribe. However, others had described him as an ambitious, self-centered, vengeful and vulnerable man who had initiated and won many fights and was intolerant of people with a different worldview.

He has been an athlete and never complained of any physical problems. However, since his forties he has had intermittent confusion accompanied by hearing voices, suggestive of possible epilepsy.

It is unclear how he reacted to the loss of many family members at a young age. Later in life he became preoccupied with doing great things and uniting all tribes and leading them. He had many emotional ups and downs and won many battles. Initially he had a small following, but gradually they grew in number. Some of them became very fanatic and fierce. After his supporters grew in number, he announced that he had a heavenly experience and started talking about receiving messages from God. He volunteered to become a mediator between some of his tribal rivals. Later he withdrew from being an active warrior, but asked his supproters to fight for a mission he had started. He became grandiose and started sending messages to his rivals that they would be better off following what he said.

His mood was not steady. After the loss of his first son, he had become very sad and isolated. He had a cabin in the woods where he would retreat during intermittent low mood, lethargy and lack of appetite. He would convince his family that he needed to pray and fast in isolation. In one episode of isolation, he started hearing voices in the cabin, which initially frightened him. Later he thought of them as God's messages.

Depending on his emotional state, the voices were at times positive and at times negative. He could differentiate them from his own thoughts. He recovered and did not hear any voices for three years. After they returned, he convinced his wife, one of his teenage cousins, and a friend that they were God's words. Gradually some other people believed him. After the loss of his wife and his uncle, he became depressed and started hearing hopeless messages again. At times he became agitated, expansive, and evasive and had an urges to start a new battle. Other times he felt elated and cheerful, and became more persuasive about his mission. He had difficulty with writing, but dictated the messages to his supporters and they made a manuscript out of them.

Physical Exam, Laboratory and Imaging Data, Allergy, Review of System, and Mental Status Exam was not available

Assessment in absentee is typically not fair. However, one might conclude that occasional isolation, fasting and sadness could be sign of depression, and that the intervals of elation, expansiveness, grandiosity, aggression, initiation of battles, paranoia and multiple marriages could be signs of mania. Mood congruent psychotic features have accompanied both episodes of his mood fluctuations at times. Intermittent severe emotional changes, confusion and hallucinations might also indicate epilepsy and postictal psychosis.

Surviving many traumas and losses might be indicative of his physical and mental strengths. Loss of many family members during childhood and being raised as an orphan by different relatives might have had an impact on his development as a righteous and self-made man. The losses could have also led to self-centered behavior, aggression, preoccupation with control, expansiveness and an intense desire for variety in satisfying his sexual needs.

Based on the information Mr. Q's diagnosis included:

Axis I: Bipolar I Disorder with psychotic features

Axis II: Cluster B personality traits

Axis III: Possible Epilepsy

Axis V: Severe; frequent losses since childhood

V: GAF had ranged from 30-80 depending on the condition

Treatment is not applicable in absentee. However, if any of the patient's descendants or relatives suffers from similar signs and symptoms, one might consider anticonvulsants not only for epilepsy but also as mood stabilizers. Lithium and neuroleptics would also have a significant benefit for bipolar disorder and psychotic features. During a depressive episode, one might transitionally add an antidepressant to help with low mood as well as impulsivity. Intensive psychotherapy to process past losses and traumas, as well as helping the individual understand his weaknesses and strengths, would be essential in recovery. Helping the tribes to understand mental illness in general and the illness of a leader in particular could have a significant impact on the community. However, some underdeveloped communities might be reluctant to question things for the sake of keeping tradition. I am optimistic though that just as developed societies have challenged sacred traditions, developing communities will eventually do the same.

Mood and Creativity and the Role of Treatment

Abstract

Objective: Many patients who suffer from a mood disorder are reluctant to follow treatment recommendations, especially pharmacological intervention. Some with an artistic temperament argue that treatment would have a negative effect on their creativity. The purpose of this article is to review the literature on mood or affective disorders, what to look for in the workup and symptom cluster to establish the diagnosis, what studies have been done on the link between the two, and the effects of treatment on creativity.

Method: The available and relevant literature on pub med was reviewed, using keywords such as "affective disorder" or "mood disorder" and "creativity." In addition to some of the standard available books in the field, a popular website was also reviewed, as noted in reference list.

Results: Episodic changes in the functioning of mind do not have a social and cultural boundary. One of the most studied spectrums of mental illness that have been associated with episodic changes is the affective or mood disorder spectrum that includes dysthymia, cyclothymia, major depression and bipolar disorder. Many studies have suggested a link between affective disorders and creativity, both of which happen to be episodic. Creative patients suffering from any of the disorders in this spectrum might question the need for treatment, either because of fear of stigma or the negative effect of the treatment on their creativity.

Conclusion: The link between creativity and mood disorder is controversial, yet clinicians agree that treatment has a positive effect on the patients' overall wellbeing and creativity.

Introduction

Episodic changes in the functioning of the mind could lead to creativity, mental illness, or both. Benjamin Rush, the father of American Psychiatry and a signer of the Declaration of Independence, had once said, "From a part of the brain preternaturally elevated, but not diseased, the mind sometimes discovers not only unusual strengths and acuteness, but certain talents it never exhibited before; talents for eloquence, poetry, music and painting, and uncommon ingenuity in several of the mechanical arts are often evolved in this state of madness"[1].

Contrary to the stigma that mental illness afflicts only socially disadvantaged, uneducated, lazy, and violent individuals, it seems that personal and social background is not a major factor in the illness of many great minds, such as Vincent Van Gogh [2], Nikolai Gogol [3], Abraham Lincoln, and Winston Churchill [4], to name a few. The purpose of this article is to review the literature on the mood or affective disorders, which is notable for episodic changes in the functioning of the mind that can be indicative of illness, creativity, or both.

Establishing Diagnosis of an Affective Disorder

The details of a comprehensive diagnostic interview and work-up to establish the diagnosis of an affective disorder can be found in major psychiatric textbooks. As an example, Hagop Akiskal, an expert on mood disorders, has described the details of a mood or affective disorder spectrum in Sadock and Kaplan's textbook of psychiatry that include dysthymia, major depression, cyclothymia, and bipolar disorder (5). What differentiates patients with affective disorder from others is that their episodic illness manifests itself with certain signs and symptoms. Instead of reviewing all of the textbook's criteria of the spectrum of affective disorders, I will try to highlight major clinical signs and symptoms and elements of the diagnostic interview and work-up in clinical practice.

While dysthymia is characterized by chronic mild sadness and pessimistic attitude for at least two years in adults, a major depressive disorder might manifest itself by persistent sadness, crying spells, loss of interest, fatigue, poor concentration, lack of self-esteem, and changes in eating habits for at least two weeks. The depressed patient might feel overwhelmed with daily activity, become irritable and argumentative, and even think of giving up on life. In severe cases, the depressed individual might lose any ability to function and become delusional or start hallucinating.

Cyclothymia might present with mood swings such as low-grade depression, agitation, or elation and impulsivity lasting a few hours to a few days, but frequently during the year. In cases of bipolar disorder, the individual might present with a manic or mixed episode with symptoms such as irritability, fidgetiness, dysphoria, high energy, no need for sleep, grandiosity, engaging in intensified simultaneous activities such as dancing, singing, drawing, writing, excessive talking and phone calls, and impulsive intimate relations. This could ultimately end in a downswing, with increased feelings of guilt, preoccupation with past unpleasant experiences, and suicidal thoughts. The symptoms might last a few days to a few weeks, or even a few months at times. In cases of psychotic experiences, individuals might have mood-congruent grandiose delusions, such as being the Savior, and having hallucinations such as seeing the "Light" or hearing messages from God or dead people. It's not unusual for these individuals to also have incongruent nihilistic delusions and hallucinations, such as the belief that the world will soon be coming to an end, based on whatever messages they believe they've been given. If left untreated, these individuals might engage in unusual and risky activities, such as sudden promiscuity, expansive business contracts, and even attacking others for perceived threats. Patients with clear-thinking processes might describe their condition as a great experience, an enjoyable chaos, or a chaotic discomfort. If artistic, these patients might express their inner turmoil through their writings, drawings or playing music. In severe cases, the expression of their talent might be too disorganized and chaotic to the point that it loses its artistic quality.

During the interview, patients might attribute their distress to life events, conflicts during upbringing, the influence of mind-altering substances and personality disorders. While these could play a role, with careful questioning and collateral information from family members, the clinician can often detect episodic changes of affect in the patient regardless of baseline personality and psychosocial events. Patients with affective disorder might be rational, calm, considerate, and productive or have personality traits of cluster B (dramatic, histrionic, manipulative, self-centered, impulsive), cluster C (avoidant, anxious, pessimistic, obsessed), and even cluster A (suspicious, eccentric and odd). Regardless of their baseline personality, the afflicted patients might feel, think, and behave differently during episodes of illness, if afflicted with an affective disorder.

Although a family history of mental illness might be denied, careful interviewing can reveal disturbances in some family members. One needs to ask about the conditions, changes, habits, and personality of blood-related family members, such as grandparents, parents, siblings, aunts, uncles, nieces, nephews and cousins. In the interview, one might detect excessive alcohol consumption, use of illicit drugs, anxiety, mood changes, ritualistic and obsessive behaviour, episodic grandiose ideas and planning, impulsivity, euphoria, frequent relationship changes, and excessive fights and arguments in the family. One needs also to ask about self-medicated approaches of family members, such as use of herbs, light boxes, and even alcohol or illicit drugs.

In terms of past psychiatric history, it's not unusual to hear about minor ups and downs of the patient, dating back to childhood or adolescence. Some might have been already treated for lack of attention span and hyperactivity as children. Some might have already seen a counselor for crying spells, behavioral changes, agitation, depression, impulsivity and rebellious behavior. Review of their medical history, especially in regard to endocrine abnormalities, seizures, head injuries, strokes, migraines and other neurological disorders, as well as a review of routine laboratory work-ups, is essential. Inquiring about past hospitalizations, medication trials, their effects and side effects, as well as psychotherapeutic treatments, are important in pinpointing a diagnosis and optimal treatment options. One needs also to ask about factors that have led to periods of stability.

In terms of mental status, patients with affective disorders might be restless, fidgety, hyperactive, or slow with psychomotor retardation. They might be withdrawn or evasive. Their speech might be rapid, expansive and loud or slowed and soft; their mood might be depressed, irritable, nervous or expansive; their affect could be congruent or incongruent, depressed, tearful or euphoric. They might have a circumstantial or tangential thought process and be preoccupied with racing, obsessive, suicidal, violent, grandiose, nihilistic and paranoid thoughts. Their perception might contain illusions and hallucinations. Their insight and judgment might be compromised.

Based on adequate information from the interview and the patient's presentation, the clinician makes a diagnosis and recommends treatment. If adequate information is not available, the clinician usually awaits resolution of possible factors, such as toxicity or other medical illnesses, job or relationship loss, lack of social support, or legal or other conflicts before making a clear diagnosis of an affective disorder.

Studies on Creativity and Affective Disorder:

Rothenberg describes creativity as an artistic ability that helps with establishing an identity as a necessary foundation for lifelong motivation (6). Nowakowska C, et al (7) compared self-reported measures of temperament and personality in a study of 49 patients with bipolar disorder, 25 with major depression, 32 creative controls, and 47 normal controls. Patients with mood disorders and creative controls had common temperamental traits. Bipolar and creative controls had the additional commonality of increased openness compared to normal controls. The study suggested underlying neurobiological commonalities between people with mood disorders and individuals involved in creative disciplines. In other words, creative individuals and patients with mood disorders had common temperamental traits.

Andreasen et al (8) compared symptom clusters in 30 writers and their relatives vs. 30 controls and their relatives. Compared to10% among the controls, about 43% of the relatives of the writers group had symptoms of mental illness, predominantly affective disorders with a tendency toward the bipolar subtype. Jamison KR. (9) investigated periods of intense creative activity and hypomania in poets, novelists, playwrights, biographers, and artists and noted that among 47 prize winning artists, 38% had been treated for affective disorders.

Ludwing (10) reviewed biographies of 1004 persons in the New York Times and noted that the rate of manic episodes was three times higher among artists compared to the entire staff (10 vs. 3%). Post (11) reviewed the biographies of British writers and noted 82 out of 100 had symptoms of at least one of the bipolar spectrum, which included bipolar psychoses, unipolar psychoses, severe depression, mild depression, brief reactive depressive traits, and cyclothymic traits.

Co-morbid cluster B and C personality disorders, substance use, impulse control disorders, attention deficit hyperactive disorder and anxiety disorders are common phenomenon in patients with bipolar disorder. Aksiakal (12) suggests that such co-morbidities might testify to the evolutionary context of affective disorders. Lara DR et al proposed a bimodal approach to understanding co-morbidity and affective disorders (13).

In a study by Simeonova et al. (14), 40 adults with bipolar disorder, 20 bipolar offspring with bipolar disorder, 20 bipolar offspring with ADHD, and 18 healthy control parents and their healthy control children completed the Barron-Welsh Art Scale (BWAS). The art scale rating of adults with bipolar disorder was 120% higher (sg.), offspring with bipolar 61% (nsg), and offspring with ADHD 40% (nsg).

Rothenberg A (15) criticizes the connection between bipolar illness and creativity and points out that sampling, methodology, presentation of results, and conclusions of the studies are inconclusive due to inadequate or absent controls, biased selection procedures, and single interviewer-experimenter bias. Despite the controversy most investigators agree with Andreasen NC and Glick ID (16) that creative individuals are most productive when their affective symptoms are under good control with treatment.

Role of Treatment

After assuring the safety and comfort of the patient, the key is to investigate etiological factors and provide treatment based on those factors. Paul McHugh considers personality, life story, behaviour and diseases, alone or in combination, as factors that affect people's mental life (17). Personality traits could be an asset, if utilized properly, and a liability if misdirected. Treatment of personality vulnerabilities is the guide to patients becoming aware of their strengths and weaknesses. Creative patients tend to value autonomy to express their talent in the way they see fit. If they work in a collaborative atmosphere, they might need to be reminded of the need for a compromise between autonomy and collegiality to avoid conflict.

In terms of personal history from a dynamic perspective, unresolved conflicts, such as traumatic experiences and developmental tasks, such as competition and connection to the same sex parent, pressure towards independence and establishing identity, might lead to symptoms in creative individuals. This, in turn, could lead to an inner suffering and a chaotic life if there is no treatment. With a supportive and reframing therapeutic approach, the inner turmoil could sublimate into artistic activity.

From a behavioural and developmental perspective, being raised in a dysfunctional family, without adequate guidance in developing healthy coping skills, can cause patients to become oppositional, act out and take risks, such as using alcohol and drugs at early age. They might even be taken advantage of and become victimized and traumatized by more disturbed people whom they trust easily. This, in turn, can lead to the development of mistrust and a confrontational attitude toward authorities, such as teachers, employers and even physicians. McHugh (17) argues that the main focus of the treatment of behavioural disturbance is interrupting the behaviours that have had a negative impact on the patient's life. Guidance in positively utilizing inner strengths becomes the next step; in the case of creative individuals, this can bring out remarkable artistic expressions.

From a biological perspective, episodic changes in creativity and mood with depressive, hypomanic, mixed, and manic symptoms, as well as symptom clusters of mood disorders in some family members, are evidence of an endogenous affective disorder, such as bipolar illness. In such cases, biological intervention, in which a balance between the least harmful and most efficient treatment is the goal, becomes necessary to keep the individual sane and yet creative. Such an approach would range from no interventions to daily visits and hospitalization. While spontaneous recovery is possible without treatment, the risk of spontaneous recurrence of symptoms is much greater if the patient is not treated. To assure compliance, it's important to educate the patient about available pharmacological treatment and the risks and benefits of treatment.

For treatment-naïve depressed patients, a trial of an SSRI is a good choice. For those who have failed SSRIs, a novel agent such as venlafaxine, bupropion, or mirtazapine are reasonable alternatives. Tricyclics such as nortriptyline, amitryptiline and imipramine or MAOIs such as phenelzine and parnate might be more effective for treatment refractory depression.

If there is an evidence of bipolarity, among the pharmacological choices, Lithium has remained the standard mood stabilizer. Schou (18) noted in a study of 24 patients with mania that Lithium attenuated or prevented recurrences of illness and increased artistic productivity in 50% of the patients, produced no change in productivity in 25%, and decreased productivity in 25%.

The severity and type of illness, individual sensitivity, and habits of the individual in utilizing manic episodes productively might explain the difference in the effect of lithium. Judd et al., (19) noted that lithium led to slowing of cognition among three out of five normal subjects. According to similar studies, discontinuation of lithium increased productivity (20) and improved memory (21). Substitution of lithium with divalproex sodium fully or partially reduced the cognitive, motivational, or creative deficits attributed to lithium in seven bipolar patients (22). Although most anticonvulsants and atypical narcoleptics are now used for management of bipolar illness, there is no data available yet on their effect on creativity and productivity.

Conclusion:

The association of creativity with affective disorders is a controversial subject. Changes in the function of the mind can lead to creativity, mental illness, or both. Many great minds have suffered from mental illness; however, romanticizing madness as a creative force is of no benefit to suffering individuals. Proper diagnosis of affective disorders, co-morbid illnesses, and psychosocial factors are very important for proper treatment. While biological intervention is key in the treatment of symptoms of illness, psychosocial interventions, such as behavioral modification, guidance, and reframing, are necessary for the treatment of behavior, temperament and life history. Creative individuals are more productive when they are treated.

References to Mood and Creativity and the Role of Treatment:

1. Quote from Benjamin Rush (1745-1813): B-Phoenix web site, June 17, 2006) http://www.angelfire.com/home/bphoenix1/creativity.html
2. Smith M. Van Gogh and lithium. Creativity and bipolar disorder: perspective of an academic psychologist. Aust N Z J Psychiatry. 1999 Dec; 33 Suppl:S120-2.

3. Witztum E, Lerner V, Kalian M. Creativity and insanity: the enigmatic medical biography of Nikolai Gogol. J Med Biogr. 2000 May;8(2):110-6.
4. Wilson OM, 'The normal' as a culture-related concept: historical considerations. Ment Health Soc. 1976;3(1-2):57-71.
5. Akiskal, Hagop, S. Mood disorders: Clinical Features, Book Chapter from Kaplan and Sadocks' Comprehensive Textbook of Psychiatry, Seventh Edition, Lippincott Williams and Wilkins, Philadelphia, PA, 2000,
6. Rothenberg A. Creativity in adolescence. Psychiatr Clin North Am. 1990 Sep;13(3):415 34.
7. Nowakowska C, Strong CM, Santosa CM, Wang PW, Ketter TA. Temperamental commonalities and differences in euthymic mood disorder patients, creative controls, and healthy controls. J Affect Disord. 2005 Mar;85(1-2):207-15.
8. Andreasen NC. Creativity and mental illness: prevalence rates in writers and their first-degree relatives. Am J Psychiatry. 1987 Oct;144(10):1288-92
9. Jamison KR. Mood disorders and patterns of creativity in British writers and artists. Psychiatry. 1989 May;52(2):125-34.
10. Ludwing (1995) reviewed biographies of 1004 persons in New York Times
11. Post F. Verbal creativity, depression and alcoholism. An investigation of one hundred American and British writers. Br J Psychiatry. 1996 May; 168(5):545-55.
12. Akiskal HS, Akiskal KK, Haykal RF, Manning JS, Connor PD. TEMPS-A: progress towards validation of a self-rated clinical version of the Temperament Evaluation of the Memphis, Pisa,

Paris, and San Diego Autoquestionnaire. J Affect Disord. 2005 Mar;85(1-2):3-16.

13. Lara DR, Pinto O, Akiskal K, Akiskal HS. Toward an integrative model of the spectrum of mood, behavioral and personality disorders based on fear and anger traits: I. Clinical implications. J Affect Disord. 2006 May 24

14. Simeonova DI, Chang KD, Strong C, Ketter TA. Creativity in familial bipolar disorder. J Psychiatr Res. 2005 Nov;39(6):623-31. Epub 2005 Mar 2.

15. Rothenberg A. Bipolar illness, creativity, and treatment. Psychiatr Q. 2001 Summer;72(2):131-47.

16. Andreasen NC, Glick ID. Bipolar affective disorder and creativity: implications and clinical management. Compr Psychiatry. 1988 May-Jun;29(3):207-17.

17. McHugh et al (Johns Hopkins website, May 16, 2006) http://www.hopkinsmedicine.org/Psychiatry/AboutUs/perspective.html

18. Schou M. Artistic productivity and lithium prophylaxis in manic-depressive illness. Br J Psychiatry. 1979 Aug;135:97-103.

19. Judd LL, Hubbard B, Janowsky DS, Huey LY, Takahashi KI.The effect of lithium carbonate on the cognitive functions of normal subjects. Arch Gen Psychiatry. 1977 Mar;34(3):355-7.

20. Shaw ED, Mann JJ, Stokes PE, Manevitz AZ. Effects of lithium carbonate on associative productivity and idiosyncrasy in bipolar outpatients. Am J Psychiatry. 1986 Sep;143(9):1166-9.

21. Kocsis JH, Shaw ED, Stokes PE, Wilner P, Elliot AS, Sikes C, Myers B, Manevitz A, Parides M. Neuropsychologic effects of lithium discontinuation. J Clin Psychopharmacol. 1993 Aug;13(4):268-75.

22. Stoll AL, Locke CA, Vuckovic A, Mayer PV. Lithium-associated cognitive and functional deficits reduced by a switch to divalproex sodium: a case series. J Clin Psychiatry. 1996 Aug;57(8):356-9.

The Patient with Recurrent Vomiting

Objective: A case study and literature review on chronic emesis or "psychogenic" vomiting

Methods: The case of patient with chronic emesis was carefully reviewed. The patient has suffered from emesis for over two years. She had been hospitalized multiple times, diagnosed with gastrointestinal illnesses as well as Chiari malformation, and undergone various surgical procedures, pharmacological, and psychosocial intervention without significant improvement. She was hospitalized and placed under constant observation. The literature on chronic emesis was carefully reviewed and summarized in table 1.

Results: After ten days of hospitalization under constant observation and step-down outpatient psychiatric care, the patient's emesis resolved. Literature review revealed that "psychogenic" emesis is not homogenous. Many cases exhibited psychiatric co-morbidity, while others did not, and such a wide gamut of therapeutic modalities were employed in their management that no generalizations can be made.

Conclusions: Although no generalization about patient population with "psychogenic" vomiting can be made, three intervention approaches exist that can be of use to every individual with the condition: 1) Interrupt the behavior; 2) Identify and neutralize factors that sustain the behavior: a) diagnose and treat concurrent illnesses, b) address the patients' life situations with appropriate counseling and/or psychotherapy in accordance with their

93

specific needs rather than with therapeutic models, c) attend to patients' temperament while identifying and correcting any motivational defects they may have towards treatment; and 3) Establish a program to extinguish habitual aspects of the behavior.

Introduction:

Somatic disturbances have a tendency to become fixed if they recur, and sometimes even if they happen only once. When psychic commotion has ceased, they linger on and the individual senses these disturbances as physical illness that recurs on the most diverse occasions (habituation reaction). Jasper (1959)

Background:

Chronic emesis has multiple etiological factors including metabolic, endocrine, and behavioral, e.g. "nervous", "psychogenic", "functional" causes, and can end in dehydration, malnutrition and even death if untreated. This paper will consider chronic emesis exclusive of anorexia and/or bulimia nervosa syndromes, and of artificially induced vomiting.

Case reports of intractable emesis range from childhood (Gonzales-Heydrich, Kerner, & Stiener, 1991) to geriatric populations (Sloan & Mizes, 1996).

Intractable vomiting is not a modern phenomenon. Van Deth and Vandereycken (1995) reviewed cases of nervous and hysterical vomiting drawn from late nineteen century, and described a group that would not fit into contemporary constructs of anorexia or bulimia nervosa, but which either resembled classical hysteria or other forms of vomiting termed "psychogenic".

Ballmer (1993) drew the distinction between physiological vomiting -- a reflex to protect the body from harmful influences, and pathological vomiting, which persists independent from such influences or causes secondary clinical consequences. He described "psychogenic" vomiting as a form of chronic pathological vomiting for which there is no medical explanation.

However, reliable distinctions between medical and psychogenic explanations for pathological vomiting are not always so readily made. Many patients with unexplained vomiting may well have a gastric vulnerability, e.g. antral hypomotility, delayed emptying, abnormal gastric electrical activity, or a lower threshold for stress-related vomiting (Lancet editorial, 1992). "Psychogenic" vomiting has often been observed with asthma, another disease that can be provoked by psychological stress. Schreir at al (1984, 1987) and Hedores (1992) postulated neurological cross-connections between the vomiting and cough centers in the medulla through which afferent vagal impulses into the cough center could activate the vomiting center.

Ballmer (1993) postulated "psychogenic" vomiting as a clinical entity, triggered by or shortly after eating, characterized by no change in weight or appetite, patient indifference, and often accompanied by the presence of family conflict and a positive family history. However, "psychogenic" vomiting has also been reported in association with a number of other psychiatric disorders (Rosenthal et al 1980; Muraoke et al, 1989).

A wide variety of therapeutic approaches have been reported and suggested for "psychogenic" vomiting (See Table 1), but we have been unable to find a unifying construct for an approach to this problem or its treatment in the literature.

We present a complicated case of chronic emesis in a young patient who had extensive medical workups and multiple hospitalizations for her condition, which ultimately came to be purely behavioral, i.e. "psychogenic" in nature. We then use this case to illustrate a systematic approach to the overall formulation and management of unexplained, intractable vomiting in particular and behavioral disorders in general.

Table 1: Case reports of Psychogenic Vomiting:

Authors	Patients	Problems	Treatment	Outcome
Rosenthal, Webb, Wruble, 1980.	24 patients (20 females, 4 males, ages 19 to 67 years) saw privately practicing gastro-enterologist. 18 patients were evaluated by clinical psychologist; 6 refused to do so. 18-month follow-up.	17% Unipolar depression 6% Briquet's syndrome 6% Bulimarexia 67% Adjustment problems without major depression 6% No evidence of psychiatric problem.	All patients told that problem was stress-related and given reassurance. Of 18 patients who agreed to a psychologist's initial evaluation, 9 went on to receive psycho-therapy and relaxation training, 5 were referred for psychiatric treatment, 2 with TMJ were referred to a dentist; and 2 refused further psychological intervention.	67% improved regardless of initial psychological evaluation, 21% had no improvement but were less concerned about their vomiting, 4% completely remitted, and 8% became worse. Unipolar depressives responded well to tricyclics, insight-oriented psychotherapy and relaxation. Those with bulimarexia or Briquet's syndrome had little or no improvement.

Haggerty & Golden, 1982	Female, age 23 years	Major depression, fainting spells, headaches, and recent marriage abusive, alcoholic husband	Medical hospitalization, IV fluids, triethylperazine, amitriptyline and individual, group, and family therapy	Symptom resolution after 3-week hospitalization and 2 month follow up
MC Danal, 1982	Female, age 30 years	Childhood trauma, abusive husband, Psychogenic vomiting	Disclosure of traumatic experiences by hypnosis	Resolution of symptoms
Stravinski, 1983	Male, age 23 years	Social phobia, Psychogenic vomiting	Exposure, social skill training, cognitive modification	Reduced anxiety and abated vomiting after 7 weeks
Golden, Janke & Haggerty, 1988	2 females, ages 26 and 27 years	Major depression, Psychogenic vomiting	Hospitalization and Amoxapine treatment	Resolution of vomiting in 1 week and improvement of depression in 2 weeks

Dura, 1988	Male, age 23 years	Psychogenic vomiting, incarcerated	Self monitoring, learned to attend to discomfort and control the behavior, heightened awareness	2-3 times daily to remission after 3 days, 1 relapse after 35 days, and remission thereafter for 6 months
Willard, Swain & Winstead, 1989	2 Females, ages 26 and 15 years	Psychogenic vomiting	Weekly insight oriented therapy, combined with group, cognitive behavioral, and family therapy for 10 weeks.	Efficacious response: 26 years old reduction of vomiting from daily to once a month, and 15 year old asymptomatic for 8 months
Muraoka et al., 1989	41 females, 19 males; ages 10 to 63 years	Psychogenic vomiting and comorbid psychiatric disorder	Hospitalization, to clarify comorbidity and pattern of vomiting	(31 conversion disorder, 21 MDD, 7 other psychiatric d/o)
Gonzales-Hydrick, Kerner & Steiner, 1991	4 females, ages 6 to 8 years	Psychogenic vomiting	Hospitalization and diagnostic clarification	3 had undiagnosed organic problems, 1 had strong psychological component

Limsila, 1996	6 children, sex and age undetermined	Psychogenic vomiting	Hospitalization, Symptom treatment, medication, psychotherapy, behavioral therapy, recreational therapy, occupational therapy, special classes, family therapy	In follow up after 20 years 5 cases had remained asymptomatic without medicine and 1 had moved to another city
Sloan & Mizes, 1996	Male, age 60 years	Psychogenic vomiting	Changing the contingency of illness behavior by rewarding independence and ignoring illness behavior	Recovered
Hsiao, Liu, Chen & Yeh, 1998	2 females, ages 22 and 50 years	Anxiety, Psychogenic vomiting	Pharmacotherapy, relaxation training, cognitive and supportive therapy	Reduced anxiety and vomiting

Case:

An 18-year-old, single, white female presented with a 2-1/2 year history of intractable vomiting, abdominal pain, and syncopal episodes, was admitted to The Johns Hopkins Eating Disorder Service for evaluation and treatment after having undergone extensive but failed medical and surgical treatments.

Her family history was notable for problematic gambling by her father, an eating disorder in a paternal aunt, and bulimia and alcohol abuse in a paternal cousin. Her birth, development, and childhood health were unremarkable. She grew up in a stable, middle class, nuclear household in which both parents worked. She repeated the first grade, and made up the lost year via home schooling. For the ninth grade, at age 15 years, she started attending a private school that she found too challenging, so she returned to public school for the tenth grade. After the onset of her illness, she -- together with her family, decided to return to home schooling until she finished high school. She had no legal, alcohol, or illicit drug use history. Her medical history was unremarkable prior to history of present illness.

At age 15 years, she first presented with a four-week history of diarrhea, which later alternated with constipation, and led to a diagnosis of irritable bowel syndrome. Two months later she developed abdominal pain and postprandial emesis. Subsequently she had multiple admissions to local hospitals and underwent extensive evaluations that included 2 abdominal ultrasounds, and abdominal MRI, hepatitis and auto-immune workups, as well as a gastric emptying scan, duodenal manometry, 4 gastro-duodenal endoscopies, 2 colonoscopies, a liver biopsy, and iminodiacetic acid radionuclide scanning. Her diagnoses included H. pylori gastritis (treated and resolved), esophagitis, eosinophilic gastritis, recurrent emesis, dehydration, transient hepatitis, and antroduodenal dysmotility consistent with chronic pseudo-obstruction. Initial radioallergosorbent test (RAST) indicated allergies to cow's milk protein, soy, and peanuts, but subsequent RAST testing was negative. Her vomiting persisted for 2.5 years, and she came to receive nourishment via NG-, G-, and J-tubes, as well as via total parentral nutrition (TPN). Tubes and lines were replaced multiple times because of malfunctioning, rupture, cellulitis, central line infection, etc. She once was observed with the tip of her central line in her mouth, which she denied. She complained of being "tired of the whole thing".

In addition to her GI symptoms, she reported recurrent syncopal episodes, that lasted from a few seconds to five minutes, sometimes in conjunction with her abdominal pain, but often without warning. EKG, a Holter-Monitor, and sleep-deprived EEG studies were negative, but neurally mediated hypotension was diagnosed via a tilt-table test. Trials of fludrocortisone and sertraline, provided no relief, and paroxetine provided partial relief.

The patient also complained of blurry, double vision and daily bitemporal headaches that were worse at night. A head MRI revealed a prominent Chiari I malformation. During surgical correction, her tonsils were clearly well below the foramen magnum. Post-operatively, the headaches improved, but the syncope and GI symptoms did not.

In the meantime, the patient's mother quit her job in order to provide care at home, and her father became distraught that no one could figure out what was wrong with her. Her frequent absence from her new school, and ultimate home schooling, marginalized her socially such that it became difficult to make new friends let alone sustain existing relationships. Her peer group gradually became limited to other chronically ill patients that she had befriended during her recurrent and protracted hospitalizations. Her sister interrupted her college education to return home to "support" the increasingly isolated patient.

Throughout the course of her illness, many child and adolescent psychiatric consultations were obtained: the patient adamantly denied binging, purging, restricting, any manipulation of her GI intake or output, and any facilitation of her vomiting. No family conflicts or secondary gains could be reliably identified that might have provoked or rewarded her continued symptoms. Therapeutic interventions ranged from keeping behavioral journals, to family therapy aimed at somehow promoting patient independence, to relaxation therapy. The patient was sent to a local partial hospitalization program for eating disorders on a psychiatric unit for three months, but her symptoms persisted necessitating multiple readmissions to the GI service, during the last of which an eating disorder consultant recommended her admission to the psychiatric inpatient Eating Disorders Unit.

On admission to the Eating Disorders Service, the patient presented as a mildly obese (body mass index = 28, at 5'6", 171#) young white female with unremarkable vital signs. She complained of vomiting, ongoing bloating, and intermittent abdominal pain. Physical examination revealed only a grade 2/6 physiologic systolic murmur, an in-place J-tube, and 3 clean sutures on her upper chest status post recent removal of a Hickman catheter. On mental status examination she was well groomed, cooperative, attentive, pleasant, in no acute distress, and had good eye contact. She spoke with regular rate, rhythm, tone, and coherence. She was euthymic, had full range of affect and intact vital sense and self-attitude, with the exception of *"la belle indifference"* she displayed with regard to her extensive medical maladies and work-up. She had no elicitable hallucinations, delusions, obsessions, compulsions, or panic/anxiety/phobic symptoms. She was awake and alert and scored 26/30 on MMSE due to poor performance on serial 7's. Her fund of general information was average, except for her familiarity with multiple psychological and medical terms. She attributed all of her problems to GI dysmotility, and said, "All I want to do is to eat normally."

The patient's Eysenck Personality Inventory scores (Neuroticism = 1, Extraversion = 13) suggested her temperament to be extremely stable but mildly extraverted, and her 20-item GHQ score of 1 (Goldberg, Anthony et al) suggested minimal subjective emotional distress – both consistent with her psychiatric presentation, her subjective symptom reports, and her statements of "tired(ness) of the whole thing".

In initially formulating this case, we thought that its most salient feature was this patient's abnormal eating behavior, which, regardless of its origins, might now be more provocative of than provoked by any ongoing GI abnormalities. We also postulated that while this patient might be/had been deriving many benefits of "the sick role", its unintended consequences were now yielding negative results. The DSM-IV translation of this formulation was Factitious disorder with physical symptoms, and Eating Disorder Not Otherwise Specified.

Upon arrival to the unit, the patient was instructed that her chronic physical symptoms had conditioned her GI tract such that it had become habituated to dysmotility, and that a gradual reconditioning of her GI tract would be required to improve her symptoms. Accordingly, the patient's tube feedings were discontinued immediately, and she was placed on a 1500 cal soft diet. In accordance with the Eating Disorders Unit protocol, all meals were consumed at the same table with all other patients with eating disorders as well as a member of the nursing staff, who stayed with them in a common area after meals. The patient was also placed on 24-hour constant observation – which she initially protested, but to which she acquiesced after being told that it was part of her protocol – in part to help prevent aspiration. The protocol also mandated that she attend all group therapy and other activity sessions with all other eating disorder patients. Her weight was monitored daily. We continued her admission medication regimen without change: ondansetron 4mg tid for emesis, and ranitidine 150mg qd for dyspepsia, and atenolol 50mg qd for neurally mediated hypotension.

At her first meal, the patient reported nausea and had emesis. She was given Ensure-Plus supplements to make up calories lost due to emesis. She had no further emesis that day; but the following morning she vomited after two forkfuls of breakfast, and vomited back Ensure, which was then substituted for breakfast, as well. Although it took 45 minutes for her to finish a soft lunch, she had no emesis. This accomplishment was met with cheers and clapping by her peers. She had no further episodes of emesis. On her third day of hospitalization, constant observation was reduced to nights only.

The patient continued to be pleasant, euthymic and to show indifference with regard to her GI condition. Her participation in group therapy was marginal, as she expressed her belief that her problem was not the same as those of other eating disorder patients. However, she readily acknowledged that her GI tract could "relearn" its natural function so that she could become symptom-free. Staff reinforced this message at meetings with family members. No explanatory interpretations for her behavior, e.g. secondary gain, psychological conflict, etc. were ever offered.

On her fifth hospital day, she was advanced to a 2,000 cal regular diet, which she tolerated without incident. Two days later, her gastroentrologist removed the J-tube. She remained asymptomatic during home visits on hospital days #11 and #12, after which she announced, "I am starting a whole new life." She was discharged to home on day #13 in good condition with normal oral intake, and without nausea or and emesis.

After discharge, the patient was seen for several weekly follow-up visits, followed by monthly visits. Ondansetron and ranitidine were gradually discontinued. Out-patient therapy has focused on counseling with regard to "here and now" structure to her days and weeks, developing and seeing through an educational plan, starting work, and resocialization with peers. During the first two months after discharge she had two fainting spells, which did not warrant ER visits, but no further emesis.

At 18-month follow-up, the patient takes only Atenolol for NMH, and otherwise has remained symptom-free. She is working, has moved away from home, and plans to attend college next semester. Her mother has returned to work, her sister has returned to her college education, and her father, while describing her recovery as a miracle, continued to gamble until he recently filed for bankruptcy. The patient has had no further emesis since her hospital discharge.

Discussion:

In this case, chronic emesis that began in association with GI pathophysiology sustained itself despite adequate treatments of the associated medical condition. That all subsequent, reasonable medical interventions failed suggested that the vomiting was "psychogenic" in origin, implying that it was ultimately "supratentorial", i.e. under the patient's control. A host of possible psychological interpretations for this patient's behavior could have been invoked, e.g. a "cry for help" for her father's gambling, or secondary gains such as receiving extra parental attention, avoidance of anxiety-provoking academic and personal challenges (school refusal, home-schooling, achievement of independence), the sick role, becoming a "fascinating" patient with an enigmatic condition that stumped the experts, etc. The patient's *"la belle indifference"* suggested a classical hysterical reaction. Observations of the patient manipulating her lines and tubes signified at least a strong behavioral and even factitious component to the maintenance of her symptoms. However, three months on a psychiatric partial hospitalization yielded no better results than dozens of admissions to pediatric GI units. In fact, this patient recovered by employing a behavioral program based only on observations and on no psychological interpretations as to their meaning.

Hence, the term "idiopathic" might be a more precise descriptor than "psychogenic" or "functional" for unexplained, intractable emesis, because it provides a more honest explanation for its mechanism, and avoids problems inherent in ascribing it to some conscious or unconscious patient motivation or dynamic that can be neither proved nor disproved, and which tend to back both the patient and the treatment team into opposite therapeutic corners. Moreover, the term "idiopathic" also allows for consideration of organic vulnerabilities, which by themselves might not be sufficient to cause this syndrome, and for simple habituation and classical conditioning -- which have nothing to do with patient motivation, as contributory factors.

Idiopathic vomiting describes neither a homogeneous group of behavioral disorders nor a homogeneous patient population. This case illustrates why each patient should be formulated on his/her own merit: many plausible pathophysiologic mechanisms could have been invoked to explain the onset of the chronic emesis, but none could explain its continuation, illustrating three fundamental points about the evolution and management of behavioral disorders in general and idiopathic vomiting in particular: 1) initiating factors may have nothing to do with sustaining factors; 2) employment of descriptors such as "psychogenic" and "functional" imply an unsubstantiated knowledge of etiologic mechanisms and motivations; and, 3) their resolution and management may not lie with either understanding or clinically "undoing" their putative cause.

This case also illustrates that a systematic and uniform approach to treatment can be applied to such a heterogeneous population: 1) interrupt the behavior; 2) identify and neutralize factors that sustain the behavior: a) diagnose and treat concurrent illnesses, b) address the patients' life situations with appropriate counseling and/or psychotherapy in accordance with their specific needs rather than with therapeutic models, c) attend to patient's temperament while identifying and correcting any motivational defects they may have toward treatment; and 3) Establish a program to extinguish habitual aspects of the behavior.

Table 1, which summarizes recent case reports on the treatment of "psychogenic" vomiting, underscores the point that it neither describes a homogenous condition nor a homogeneous patient population: many cases exhibited psychiatric co-morbidity, while others did not, and as such a wide gamut of therapeutic modalities were employed in their management that no generalizations can be made.

In this case, we first interrupted the patient's behavior by limiting caloric intake to only that which could be taken orally, putting her on 24-hour constant observation, and ultimately removing her tubes. The importance of 24-hour supervision to interrupt intractable behavior cannot be overstated. We next surveyed four factors which could be sustaining her behavior: a complete GI work-up proved negative, detailed mental status examinations revealed no significant psychopathological symptoms, General Health Questionnaire revealed no evidence of great subjective distress, Eysenck Personality Inventory revealed no obvious temperamental vulnerabilities, and a review of her psychosocial situation revealed problems, but no obvious conflicts. We finally established a structural behavioral program comprised of gradual, regimented increases in oral intake, nutrition and menu education, peer group therapy to provide feedback and serve as a reservoir of encouragement and moral support, and individual counseling to guide her and her family in orderly steps to re-assume their respective home, educational, and occupational roles.

The approach to behavioral disorders in general and to this case of idiopathic vomiting in particular is entirely parsimonious with The Lancet editorial position (1992) that although patients with unexplained vomiting may be experiencing high level of stress or have a lower threshold for vomiting, idiopathic vomiting is to be considered only after other etiologies have been excluded (see also Gonzalez-Heydrich et al, 1991): moreover, even "hysterical" patients can develop primary or secondary illnesses, just as sick patient can develop 'hysterical' symptoms as artifact, e.g. seizure patient with pseudo seizures Bowman and Markand (1999). The fact of medical or psychiatric co-morbidity does not alter the ultimate behavioral management of these disorders. However, co-morbidities must be compensated before relying upon a behavioral program. In this case, the patient's GI and CNS conditions had been adequately diagnosed and treated before implementing a behavioral plan.

References to Psychogenic Vomiting:

1. Bowman ES, Markand ON. The contribution of life events to pseudoseizure occurrence in adults. Bull Menninger Clin 1999 Winter; 63(1): 70-88

2. Limsila P. Psychogenic vomiting 1976-1981, follow-up treatment results up to 1996. J Med Assoc Thai 1998 Feb; 81(2): 117-24

3. Gonzalez-Heydrich J, Kerner JA Jr, Steiner H. Testing the psychogenic vomiting diagnosis. Four pediatric patients. Am J Dis Child 1991 Aug; 145(8): 913-6.

4. Stravynski A. Behavioral treatment of psychogenic vomiting in the context of social phobia. J Nerv Ment Dis 1983 Jul; 171(7): 448-51

5. Muraoka M, Mine K, Matsumoto K, Nakai Y, Nakagawa T. Psychogenic vomiting: the relation between patterns of vomiting and psychiatric diagnoses. Gut 1990 May; 31(5): 526-8

6. Ballmer PE. Persistent vomiting Schweiz Med Wochenschr 1993 Apr 17; 123(15): 687-93 (Article in German)

7. McHugh PR, Slavney PR. The Perspectives of Psychiatry, second edition, The Johns Hopkins University Press, Baltimore, 1983

8. Editorial, Psychogenic vomiting--a disorder of gastrointestinal motility? Lancet. 1992 Feb 1; 339(8788): 279.

9. Hederos CA, Psychogenic vomiting. Lancet. 1992 May 16, 339(8803): 1228.

10. Korkina MV, Marilov VV, [Variants of psychosomatic personality development in diseases of the gastrointestinal tract, Zh Nevropatol Psikhiatr Im S S Korsakova. 1995; 95(6): 43-7. Russian article.

11. Van Deth R, Vandereycken W; Was late-nineteenth-century nervous vomiting an early variant of bulimia nervosa? Hist Psychiatry. 1995 Sep; 6(23 Pt 3): 333-47.

12. Barth N, Riegels M, Heberbrand J, Remschmidt H. ["Cyclic vomiting" in childhood and adolescence], Z Kinder Jugendpsychiatr Psychother. 2000 May; 28(2): 109-17. Review. German.

13. Rosenthal RH, Webb WL, Wruble LD. Diagnosis and management of persistent psychogenic vomiting. Psychosomatics. 1980 Sep; 21(9): 722-30.

14. Haggerty JJ Jr, Golden RN. Psychogenic vomiting associated with depression. Psychosomatics. 1982 Jan; 23(1): 91-5.

15. McDanal CE. Psychogenic vomiting and depression. Psychosomatics. 1982 Sep; 23(9): 957-8.

16. Stravynski A. Behavioral treatment of psychogenic vomiting in the context of social phobia. J Nerv Ment Dis. 1983 Jul; 171(7): 448-51.

17. Golden RN, Janke I, Haggerty JJ Jr, Amoxapine treatment of psychogenic vomiting and depression. Psychosomatics. 1988 summer; 29(3): 352-4. No abstract available.

18. Dura JR. Successful treatment of chronic psychogenic vomiting by self-monitoring. Psychol Rep. 1988 Feb; 62(1): 239-42.

19. Willard SG, Swain BS, Winstead DK. A treatment strategy for psychogenic vomiting. Psychiatr Med. 1989; 7(3): 59-73.

20. Limsila P. Psychogenic vomiting 1976-1981, follow-up treatment results up to 1996. J Med Assoc Thai. 1998 Feb; 81(2): 117-24.

21. Hsiao CC, Liu CY, Chen CK, Yeh SS. Psychogenic vomiting: report of two cases. Changgeng Yi Xue Za Zhi. 1998 Dec; 21(4): 514-20.

22. Sloan DM, Mizes JS. The use of contingency management in the treatment of a geriatric nursing home patient with psychogenic vomiting. J Behav Ther Exp Psychiatry. 1996 Mar;27(1):57-65.

23. Schreir L, Curder RM, Saigal V. The vomiting asthmatic. Americal Allergy; 1984; 53:42-44.

24. Schreir L, Curder RM, Saigal V. Vomiting as a dominant symptom of asthma. Americal Allergy; 1987; 58:118-20.